The Adventurous Traveler's Guide to Health

The Adventurous Traveler's Guide to Health

CHRISTOPHER SANFORD, M.D.

UNIVERSITY OF WASHINGTON PRESS   Seattle and London

© 2008 by the University of Washington Press
Printed in the United States of America
Designed by Ashley Saleeba
13 12 11 10 09 08   5 4 3 2 1

UNIVERSITY OF WASHINGTON PRESS
PO Box 50096, Seattle, WA 98145
www.washington.edu/uwpress

LIBRARY OF CONGRESS CATALOGING-IN-PUBLICATION DATA
Sanford, Christopher.
The adventurous traveler's guide to health / Christopher Sanford.
p.   cm.
Includes bibliographical references and index.
ISBN 978-0-295-98808-5 (pbk. : alk. paper)
1. Travel—Health aspects—Handbooks, manuals, etc.   I. Title.
RA783.5.S26   2007
613.6'8—dc22   2007039032

The paper used in this publication is acid-free and 90 percent recycled
from at least 50 percent post-consumer waste. It meets the minimum
requirements of American National Standard for Information Sciences—
Permanence of Paper for Printed Library Materials, ANSI Z39.48–1984.

To my parents

Contents

Acknowledgments

I would like to thank Dr. Elaine Jong of the University of Washington, who first pulled me into the world of travel medicine; Drs. Jennifer Leaning and Richard Cash of the Harvard School of Public Health for their support and editorial wisdom; Jacqueline Ettinger, Mary Ribesky, Beth Fuget, Nanette Pyne, Pat Soden, and Ashley Saleeba of University of Washington Press for their many sage suggestions; Drs. David O. Freedman and Eduardo Gotuzzo for hosting the Gorgas Course in Clinical Tropical Medicine in Lima, Peru; my ER consultant Dr. Mike Peterson; my pulmonology consultant Dr. Gordon Rubenfeld; my pediatrics consultants Drs. Jean Haulman, Sheila Mackell, Jonathan Spector, and Doug Diekema; my malaria consultants Dr. Alan Magill and Jay Keystone; my high-altitude consultants Drs. Jim Litch and Rachel Bishop; my infectious disease consultant Dr. Wes Van Voorhis; my motor vehicle safety consultant Dr. Charles Mock; my rabies consultant Dr. Henry Wilde; my gastroenterology consultant Dr. Bradley A. Connor; my neurosurgery consultant Dr. Sanford Wright; my entomology consultants Andy Spielman, Junko Yasuoka, Michael Reddy, and Scott Carroll; my Brit doc consultant Dr. Andrew Moscrop; my family practice consultants Dr. Bill Stauffer and Dr. Mike Werner; my geography consultants Jonathan Mayer and Craig Jeffrey; my corporate medicine consultant Dr. Richard Weller; my jet health consultant Dr. Michael Muhm; my security consultant Joel McNamara; my nurse practitioner consultants Britt Murphy and Annie Terry; my loyal and long-suffering readers Ondi Lingenfelter, Barbara Baker, Erik Christensen, and Ina Chang; my orthopedic consultant Dr. Bill Thieme; my brother Ren for first pointing out to me that coconut trees can present a threat to tourists' well-being; my brother Curt for translating Spanish; my wife Sallie for love, sanity, and perspective; my sons Nathaniel and Henry for reminding me that it's permissible—indeed wise—to do something just for fun-ness.

Author's Note

WHAT THIS BOOK IS NOT

This guide is not intended to replace your visit to a pre-travel provider, who will evaluate your personal health history, itinerary, and planned activities, then make specific recommendations. Rather the ambition of this guide is to prepare you for your consultation with your pre-travel provider and forearm you regarding strategies that will keep you fit during your travels.

Travel medicine, like other fields of medicine, is an ever-changing discipline. Recommendations change over time as new studies are incorporated into the body of knowledge on which we base our advice. I have attempted to offer all treatment protocols with the latest available information, but readers should consult their own physicians for the most up-to-date recommendations. You should confirm all drug doses, interactions with other drugs, and possible side effects with your pre-travel provider. Additionally, this is a guide, not a comprehensive medical text; discussion of many topics is necessarily summary. Those readers seeking a more in-depth discussion of topics pertinent to travel medicine should look to any of the many textbooks of travel medicine listed in the bibliography.

The Adventurous Traveler's Guide to Health

Introduction

The purpose of this guide is to reduce your risk of illness and injury while traveling abroad. Although the focus is on the developing world, much of this advice applies to travel in the industrialized world as well. My emphasis is on common illnesses and injuries. As titillating as shark bites and lightning strikes may be, they don't make it onto my radar; if something occurs less frequently than one-in-a-million, it probably isn't going to happen to you. I am concerned with common problems: car crashes, travelers' diarrhea, hepatitis A.

One theme of this work is that noninfectious threats to international travelers are generally underemphasized by pre-travel providers and underappreciated by travelers. Another key theme is that these threats are not random; prudent precautions can reduce risk. Reading through travel health literature, I am struck again and again by the fact that risk is less determined by where you go than by what you do. It is only a slight overstatement to say that there are not risky destinations, but only risky travelers.

And why should you travel to the developing world? Why should you voluntarily visit a land with sketchy plumbing and dodgy roads? The lure of these countries is difficult to explain.

Those of us who gravitate toward travel in the poorer regions of the world (and our numbers are large: every year over 75 million people travel from industrialized nations to the developing world) experience equal parts adrenaline and wonder. Travel to the developing world will elevate the mundane into the realm of the considered; it will show you what is left of you when you remove routine and reflex.

It is important, I think, to realize that our own corner of the world is not representative; most of us who live in North America and Western Europe are, in fact, wealthy and lucky. For many of us, travel to the developing world is a life-changing experience. During our travels we may come to appreciate, in a manner that would be impossible had we remained within the wealthy nations, the vast magnitude of global inequalities; after our return we may newly appreciate our usual environs.

People visit the developing world for myriad reasons: to study, to serve, to recreate, to conduct business, to visit the land of their forebears. Regardless of your motivation, a few precautions will minimize the risk of illness or injury during your travels; hence my book.

TRAVEL MEDICINE Q & A

Q What do you mean by "the developing world"?

A This is an economic term, not a geographic one; it refers to nations that are poor. The US, Canada, Western Europe, Australia, New Zealand, Japan, and Singapore are considered to be developed countries; most nations in Africa, Latin America, and Asia are developing. There is a wide range of affluence within all nations, poor and wealthy alike, but the average income in developing nations is below a given threshold.

Q **Are all these countries really developing?**

A No. It's just a term. Some are developing, some are stable, in some things are getting worse. These countries are also known as low-income countries, or, formerly, the third world.

Q **Is "travel medicine" really a medical specialty or did you just make that up?**

A It exists. It is a new specialty, extant for approximately thirty years. It has been defined as "the discipline devoted to the maintenance of the health of international travelers through health promotion and disease prevention." * It is an interdisciplinary field, drawing on the fields of infectious disease, public health, preventative medicine, and a host of other medical specialties and subspecialties.

Q **Can any medical provider give me advice regarding travel medicine?**

A No. Most medical providers do not see a sufficient number of international travelers to be proficient on travel medicine. You want to see someone who sees international travelers on a regular basis.

Q **How do I find a pre-travel provider?**

A Both the International Society of Travel Medicine (ISTM) and

*This definition is from *Travel Medicine*, J.S. Keystone, et al., eds. (Edinburgh: Mosby, 2004), chapter 1.

the American Society of Tropical Medicine and Hygiene (ASTMH) maintain a list of travel clinics on their web sites: *www.istm.org*, *www.astmh.org*. Many US universities have travel clinics; some see students only, some see anyone.

Q Two or more of us have the same itinerary. Can we see the pre-travel provider at the same time and save money?

A Some travel clinics offer a discount if more than one traveler with the same itinerary is seen at the same time. However, you should be aware that personal questions—regarding past medical history, most recent menstrual period, use of birth control, medications, etc.—will be asked. If you're not comfortable answering these questions in front of your travel companions, best see your pre-travel provider one-on-one.

Q How long before our trip do we need to see the travel clinic?

A We like a month to six weeks if we can get it. Most vaccines take about two weeks to kick in (phrasing this more formally, the antibody response initiated by vaccines requires approximately two weeks to attain protective levels). A few vaccine series are given over four weeks. Another advantage of being seen at least a month prior to your departure is that you have time for a pre-travel trial of medications with potential for side effects, such as those that prevent malaria, while you are still in-country. However, travel clinics will see travelers at any time prior to their trip.

1 **Overview**

RISKS TO INTERNATIONAL TRAVELERS

~~~~~~

THE BOTTOM LINE

Seeing a pre-travel provider can markedly reduce your odds of illness and injury while abroad. A pre-travel provider is a health professional—usually a physician, nurse practitioner, physician assistant, or nurse—with expertise in the health issues of international travelers. During the pre-travel encounter your provider will evaluate you and your itinerary, then make recommendations concerning vaccines and medications, and give advice on reducing your risk of illness and accident while abroad.

~~~~~~

THE PRE-TRAVEL ENCOUNTER

You and your pre-travel provider have a number of topics to discuss during the pre-travel encounter:

+ Your past medical history, including:
    · medications
    · allergies

- surgeries
- hospitalizations
- (for women) birth control/possibility of pregnancy
- immunization history—take your immunization record to the travel clinic if you possibly can!
- prior antimalarial use

+ Itinerary
  - where and when you're going
  - your planned activities
  - type of accommodation (hostels, camping, hotels, or private home)

+ Immunizations
  - which immunizations the provider advises for this trip
  - which immunizations, if you can't afford all of them, are most important

+ Malaria
  - where malaria is and is not present in countries you will be visiting
  - personal protection measures, i.e., minimizing bug bites (which include DEET to skin, permethrin to clothes, and sleeping under a bed net)
  - medication options (for chloroquine-sensitive and chloroquine-resistant regions); pros and cons, including cost, of each

+ Travelers' diarrhea
  - dietary choices to minimize risk (this shouldn't take too long, as there is not much evidence that cautious food choice reduces your risk of diarrhea)
  - pros and cons of antibiotic self-treatment for travelers' diarrhea
  - the different available medication

+ Urban medicine: seat belts, helmets, crime, and security

- Special topics, if your itinerary so necessitates: high-altitude illness, scuba diving
- Emergency medical evacuation insurance
- How to contact the travel clinic when you're out of the country (usually by e-mail)
- Follow-up screening after your trip, if needed

Signs That Your Pre-Travel Provider May Be Suboptimal

- Does whole pre-travel encounter in under five minutes.

- Does not ask you about the topics listed above, including information about your allergies, prior experiences with antimalarials, past immunizations, current medications, etc.

- Recommends a sulfa-based drug for carry-along self-treatment of travelers' diarrhea.

- Recommends chloroquine to prevent malaria in a country other than those listed under "Chloroquine-Sensitive Countries" in chapter 3.

- Recommends yellow fever vaccine for any region other than the two discussed in chapter 2.

- Recommends gamma globulin, not hepatitis A vaccine, for someone with an intact immune system over one year of age.

If you're going to a country with malaria, try to leave the pre-travel provider's office with map in hand that shows where malaria is and where it is not.

Travelers to the developing world should consider purchasing evacuation insurance. Emergent medical evacuation to the developed world via jet is extraordinarily pricey, about US $50,000–100,000. There are a number of companies and organizations that provide emergency medical evacuation insurance; these include International SOS, MedAire, MEDEX, and Divers Alert Network (DAN). You pay a fee up front, and if emergent evacuation is required, the company flies you to an appropriate medical facility without additional charge.

Also, if you have health insurance, phone the member services department prior to your departure, and ask what they cover and what they do not. Some plans will cover you when you travel abroad; some do not. Sometimes the ones that do will ask you to bring back any receipts for medical care and they will reimburse you. Every plan is different. This is much easier to research from your country of origin prior to your trip. If you fall ill and have difficulty researching your health insurance situation due to spotty or absent telephone or Internet access, you'll kick yourself if you haven't done some advance planning.

2 Immunizations

ROUTINE, REQUIRED, RECOMMENDED

~~~~~~

THE BOTTOM LINE

+ You should be current on the usual "domestic" vaccines, including tetanus.

+ Hepatitis A and influenza are the most important vaccines for international travelers.

+ Vaccination for hepatitis B is a good idea for almost every traveler.

+ Vaccination for yellow fever is recommended for travel to most countries in tropical South America and tropical Africa; for many it is required.

+ Depending on your itinerary, duration of stay, and planned activities, other vaccines may be recommended.

~~~~~~

It is convenient to view each vaccine as falling into one of three categories: routine, required, or recommended.

ROUTINE IMMUNIZATIONS

Although most people do not associate "domestic" vaccines with international travel, in the big scheme of things these vaccines probably provide more protection to travelers than do "travel" vaccines. It is prudent for the international traveler to remain current on all standard vaccines. The current schedule of recommended vaccines for adults is posted at the CDC web site: *http://www.cdc.gov/.* Each is discussed below.

TETANUS, DIPHTHERIA, PERTUSSIS

Assuming you received the standard tetanus, diphtheria, and pertussis (DTaP) series as a child, you should get a tetanus shot every ten years. Historically, in the US, this is given as a "dip-tet," or "Td," which provides protection against tetanus and diphtheria. In 2005 a new combination vaccine, "Tdap," was released on the US market; it covers pertussis as well. In the 1990s large outbreaks of diphtheria occurred in Russia, the independent countries of the former Soviet Union, and elsewhere. Adults between the ages of 19 and 64 should substitute Tdap for one booster dose of Td.

MEASLES, MUMPS, RUBELLA (MMR)

All three of these diseases are far more common in the developing world. In the US there are fewer than 100 cases of measles per year; in the developing world there are over 10 million cases each year. Although deaths from measles dropped an estimated 60% between 1999 and 2005, there were still approximately 345,000 deaths from measles in 2005.

Those born in or after 1957 require immunization for MMR. The first dose is usually administered at about fifteen months.

A second dose, separated from the first by at least four weeks, is advised for all international travelers. Most US colleges and universities will not allow students to enroll until they have received a second dose of MMR (or demonstrate protection via a blood test). The CDC (Centers for Disease Control and Prevention) does not recommend vaccination for those born prior to 1957, as they are presumed to have immunity to these illnesses.

POLIO

Polio is not yet eradicated. A decades-long campaign coordinated by the World Health Organization (WHO) has come close to eliminating polio in most of the world. There were fewer than 500 cases in 2001, the fewest ever recorded. However, between 2002 and 2005 polio spread from six countries to an additional twenty-one countries. Transmission is ongoing in several countries in Africa, the Indian subcontinent (India, Pakistan, and Bangladesh), and Indonesia.

For adults who received the usual childhood series (either oral or injection), a single polio booster is advised; further boosters are not necessary. (Note: oral polio—"the sugar cube"—is no longer available in the US; in the US all polio immunization is given via injection.)

HEPATITIS A

Hepatitis A is the most common vaccine-preventable illness of travelers. It is caused by a virus that is spread by contaminated food and water. (In medical parlance, this route of spread is known by the rather unsettling term "fecal-oral transmission.")

Hepatitis A is a relatively mild illness in children but will land an adult in bed for several weeks; in those above age forty it carries a 2% death rate. Even in those who survive, it's not pleasant. Your skin and sclerae (the whites of your eyes) turn an alarming yellow-orange ("jaundice"). The discoloration of the skin is more difficult to detect in dark-skinned people, but the change in color of the sclerae is evident in everyone. Additionally, you develop nausea, belly pain, sweats, and general misery. You can get it only once, but for people who've been through it, once is one time too many. The vaccine is by far the preferable option.

The hepatitis A vaccine series is simple: two shots, at least six months apart. The duration of immunity to hepatitis A following this vaccine series appears to be lifelong.

Myths Regarding Hepatitis A

"It's better to get the disease than the vaccine; that way I'll have 'natural immunity.'"

No. For openers, if you're over forty and you're in the 2% that die from hepatitis A, whatever immunity you do or do not develop will be moot. Additionally, there is no evidence that protection from having had hepatitis A is in any way superior to protection from the vaccine.

"If I choose my food and drink with caution, I'll be okay."

Hepatitis A is common throughout the developing world, and you can't tell by looking at food and water whether it's safe or contaminated. The same strategies that may reduce your risk of travelers' diarrhea may reduce your risk of hepatitis A, but not to the point that you want to pass on the vaccine.

"I was born in the developing world so I'm probably protected."

There is some truth to this claim. Indeed, many people born in the developing world have had this illness, most commonly during childhood, and are protected. However, given that many people from the developing world are not protected, assuming that someone is protected is risky. People born in the developing world should either:

+ receive an antibody blood test to see if they have protection, and get the vaccine series if they do not, or
+ simply get the vaccine series.

"It's not required so it must not be important."

"Not required" doesn't mean "not advised." Hepatitis A is over a thousand times more common in international travelers than yellow fever, for which vaccination is required to enter some countries. You should base your choice of vaccines on what diseases your travel places you at risk for, not on what is required.

"I'm leaving in less than two weeks. I've read that hepatitis A vaccine takes two weeks to kick in, so I'll get gamma globulin instead."

That used to be the recommendation, but physicians now realize that even if you get your first hepatitis A vaccine dose *on the way to the airport* to fly to the developing world, you'll be protected. It works like this: After receiving the first hepatitis A immunization your body does indeed require about two weeks to develop protective antibodies (the specific molecules that your body manufactures, in response to a vaccine or infectious organism, that prevent a disease). However, hepatitis A has a minimum incubation period of two weeks, so even if you have the bad luck to be exposed to hepatitis A during your first meal abroad, a race then occurs between the incubation of the disease and the formation of antibodies. Antibodies form more quickly, so you do not get the illness.

After the first immunization for hepatitis A you are protected for only six to twelve months. You should get the second and final shot of the series six months after the first, which extends your protection for life. (Gamma globulin, which was given for protection from hepatitis A prior to hepatitis A vaccine coming onto the US market in 1995, only provides protection for a few months.)

HEPATITIS B

While more rare than hepatitis A in travelers, hepatitis B is a more serious illness, and vaccination for this disease should be considered by almost every traveler. Unlike hepatitis A, which is spread by contaminated food and water, hepatitis B is transmitted by blood and sex. In addition to having more severe symptoms and lasting for a longer duration, hepatitis B often, unlike hepatitis A, develops into a lifelong carrier state, with significant risk of liver failure.

Significantly, some long-stay travelers who report no potential risks for acquiring hepatitis B (no new partners in their sex lives, no needle pokes or tattoos) do periodically acquire this disease. Possibly the virus is entering those who lack apparent risk factors via breaks in the skin that are too small to notice. Medical or dental procedures utilizing contaminated instruments can also spread hepatitis B.

The vaccine series consists of three shots. You should receive the second and third 1 and 6 months after the first. (Or, in vaccine lingo, you get the shots at time 0, 1, and 6 months.) Protection is lifelong; there is no need for booster shots.

The routine use of hepatitis B vaccine in infants has been recommended in the US since 1991.

If you cannot receive the hepatitis B series utilizing the usual schedule because your departure is less than six months away, you can employ an "accelerated" series schedule. In the accelerated series schedule you get three shots of hepatitis B prior to your trip (on days 0, 7, and 14 to 28), then a fourth shot one year after the first. After the first three, you have most but not all of the protection that you would receive if you had had the three injections by the usual schedule; when you get the fourth at one year after the first, you are thereafter as fully protected as though you had employed the usual schedule.

There is also an accelerated schedule for Twinrix (see below), consisting of four shots, given at days 0, 7, and 21, and one year.

If you are receiving hepatitis A only, you do not need to use an accelerated series because one injection provides protection for six to twelve months.

Twinrix

There is a combination hepatitis A + hepatitis B immunization product on the market called Twinrix. This consists of three shots, at time 0, 1 month, and 6 months. Its benefits are that it's a little cheaper than getting hepatitis A and B vaccines separately, and you receive three shots as opposed to the five that you would get if you received the hepatitis A and B series separately.

INFLUENZA

Influenza, as anyone who has had it can tell you, is not just a "bad cold." It is a severe illness that lands the average victim in bed for a couple of weeks. The worldwide influenza pandemic of 1918–19 killed an estimated 50 million people; currently influenza kills 36,000 people every year in the US alone.

Travelers get influenza more frequently than do people who stay home. Additionally, travelers are more prone to acquiring this "off-season." In the US the influenza season is October to April. South of the equator, e.g., in Australia, this is exactly six months off: April to October. And near the equator there is no seasonality; it occurs sporadically throughout the year.

Influenza is common. A Swiss study found that international travelers developed influenza at a rate of one case for every 100 person-months abroad. Given that flu vaccine is inexpensive and has minimal side effects, this immunization should be considered for virtually every traveler, even if it is off-season in your country of origin. (However, it can be difficult to find during the off-season.)

VARICELLA (CHICKENPOX)

Chickenpox is usually a mild to moderately severe illness in children; it is usually more severe in adults. If you've ever had chickenpox, you are immune for life. However, if you are not sure if you've had chickenpox, you should either receive the vaccine or get a blood test to check for immunity. (Many people who do not recall a history of chickenpox are indeed immune; they probably had cases as children so mild that the illness was not recognized as chickenpox by their parents.)

Interestingly, chickenpox has a different age distribution in different regions. In temperate countries (e.g., the US), it is primarily a pediatric illness, but for unknown reasons in the tropics it is primarily an illness of young adults.

Vaccine schedule: Children between one and twelve years old should receive two doses at least twelve weeks apart; travelers thirteen years and older years require two shots separated by at least four weeks. If you only have time for one of the two doses prior to your departure, you will have some protection against this illness, but not as much as is provided by the full series. Note: As of summer 2006, forty-six US states require varicella vaccine for public school entry in children under thirteen.

PNEUMOCOCCAL DISEASE

An immunization for pneumococcal disease (pneumococcal polysaccharide vaccine [PPV]) is advised for everyone over the age of sixty-five; it is recommended in people under sixty-five who have certain chronic medical conditions including heart disease, lung disease, and diabetes. Usually only one immunization for life is advised; a second dose is advised for people aged sixty-five and older who received their first dose when they were under sixty-five, if more than five years have passed since the first dose, or for people with certain chronic medical conditions including HIV/AIDS and sickle cell anemia.

HAEMOPHILUS INFLUENZAE

Children should be current on Hib (Haemophilus influenzae) vaccine. Children over the age of five do not need Hib vaccine unless they have certain medical conditions including HIV/AIDS and sickle cell anemia.

FLU Q & A

Q What's the difference between seasonal flu and pandemic flu?

A Seasonal flu occurs every year. Pandemic flu occurs infrequently (most recently in 1968–69) and is associated with a higher-than-usual rate of illness and death.

Q **What countries have had human cases of avian flu?**

A Between 2003 and February 2008, there have been 371 cases of bird flu, resulting in 235 deaths. Cases have been reported (in decreasing frequency of number of cases per country) in Indonesia, Vietnam, Egypt, Thailand, China, Turkey, Azerbaijan, Cambodia, Iraq, Laos, Nigeria, and Djibouti. For more current information on avian influenza, see the WHO site: *http://www.who .int/csr/disease/avian_influenza/country/cases_table_2007_09_10/en/ index.html*

Q **I'm thinking of visiting a country with ongoing avian influenza transmission. Should I go?**

Avian Influenza (a.k.a. Bird Flu)

Avian influenza is caused by viruses that ordinarily only infect birds. However, since 1997, avian influenza viruses have infected a small number of people. Among the avian influenza viruses that have infected people since 1997, "H5N1" has been the most common. One reason that the numbers of those affected remains relatively low is that sustained human-to-human transmission has not occurred. The odds of avian influenza viruses mutating such that person-to-person transmission occurs are unknown.

A The CDC does not currently recommend that travelers avoid any country because of avian influenza. They do advise that travelers avoid handling live or dead birds or surfaces that might be contaminated with bird secretions or feces. Additionally, travelers should avoid poultry farms and bird markets in countries with ongoing transmission.

Q What is the risk of bird flu to the international traveler?

A It appears to be minuscule. The majority of people who contract bird flu are those who have close and ongoing contact with birds, such as chicken farmers and duck vendors.

Q What are the symptoms of bird flu infection in humans?

A Symptoms range from typical influenza symptoms—fever, muscle aches, cough—to severe respiratory illness and other life-threatening complications.

Q Can I be immunized for bird flu?

A As of January 2008 there are no vaccines on the market. It is thought that vaccine will probably not be available early in a pandemic, should one occur.

Q Are poultry and eggs safe to eat in countries with ongoing avian influenza transmission?

A Yes, if well cooked.

Q Are there any measures that might reduce my risk of this illness?

A Frequent hand washing with soap and water, or an alcohol-based gel, probably reduces risk.

Q **Should I take an antiviral medication such as Tamiflu (oseltamivir) with me when I travel to a country with ongoing bird flu transmission?**

A The benefit of Tamiflu for bird flu is unknown. Some travel medicine providers feel that it's reasonable to carry a course of Tamiflu when you travel in countries endemic for bird flu. My thought is that it's difficult for the traveler to discern if fever and aches are due to influenza or something else; I don't routinely advise carrying it.

Q **Just how worried should I be about bird flu?**

A Influenza pandemics—worse than usual flu seasons—tend to occur three or four times per century. During the twentieth century, three pandemics occurred, in 1918–19, 1957–58, and 1968–69. There will certainly be more in the future. Of note, the most severe pandemic, which occurred in 1918–19, was caused by an avian influenza virus that mutated such that it was easily transmitted between people. But the timing of the next epidemic, and whether its cause will be a traditional human influenza virus or an avian influenza virus, are unknown.

HUMAN PAPILLOMA VIRUS (HPV)

Human papilloma viruses are transmitted by sexual contact. A majority of cases resolve without treatment, but many people with HPV develop genital warts; additionally, over 99% of cancers of the cervix are caused by HPV. Although over thirty strains of

HPV are sexually transmitted, types 6 and 11 cause 90% of genital warts, and types 16 and 18 cause 70% of cervical cancer. HPV is common: it is estimated that 80% of sexually active men and women will acquire HPV infection at some point in their lives.

In June 2006 the US Food and Drug Administration (FDA) approved a vaccine for HPV that protects against strains 6, 11, 16, and 18, for females between the ages of nine and twenty-six years. The recommended schedule is to receive three doses: a second dose one to two months after the first, then a final dose six months after the first. The duration of protection is unknown but appears to be at least four years. Initial data indicate that the vaccine offers a high level of protection. The vaccine is expensive: about $360 for three doses. Currently the vaccine is only approved for use in females, but given that HPV is also linked to genital warts and malignancies of the penis and rectum in men, it may be approved for use in men in the future. Studies in men are currently being conducted.

Women who receive the vaccine should continue to receive pap smears. No testing for HPV is available for men.

REQUIRED IMMUNIZATIONS

YELLOW FEVER

Yellow fever is caused by a virus that is spread by mosquitoes. In 1793 an epidemic in Philadelphia killed between one-tenth and one-fifth of its inhabitants; those who fled town included then-president George Washington. Yellow fever is now absent from North America, but it remains endemic in much of tropical South America and tropical Africa (see maps 1 and 2).

Yellow fever is serious; in some outbreaks it kills half its victims. Symptoms are jaundice (hence its moniker), nausea, vomiting, fevers, and achiness. Once someone develops yellow fever, there is no cure. Treatment is "supportive" (physicians' buzz phrase for making patients as comfortable as possible and hoping they get well).

The CDC website states: "Four of the five cases of yellow fever among travelers from the United States and Europe in 1996–2002 were exposed in South America. All five cases were fatal and occurred among unvaccinated travelers."

The current recommendation is that someone traveling to any endemic region be vaccinated once every ten years. Many countries located in endemic regions will turn away an arrival at the airport if that traveler cannot show proof of vaccination. Additionally, many countries require evidence of yellow fever vaccination in travelers who are arriving from countries in which yellow fever is endemic, whether or not yellow fever is present in the country that the traveler is trying to enter. A list of every nation's yellow fever requirements is available at: http://www.cdc.gov. You should keep your vaccination record with your passport so that it is easily accessible at customs.

Recently, a very rare side effect of yellow fever vaccine was recognized. A small number of recipients of this vaccine will develop symptoms similar to yellow fever; this reaction has a high fatality rate. The risk of this is highest in the elderly: in those over sixty-five years old, the risk is estimated to be one in 50,000. (With the exception of vaccination for yellow fever, elderly travelers do not have a higher rate of adverse effects from vaccines than do younger travelers.) Because yellow fever is a life-threatening disease, the CDC continues to recommend that people who will be visiting areas with yellow fever receive the vaccine. However, if you're visiting a country with yellow fever but are not going to an area within that country where yellow fever is transmitted, your pre-travel provider can write an exemption letter. This letter, best

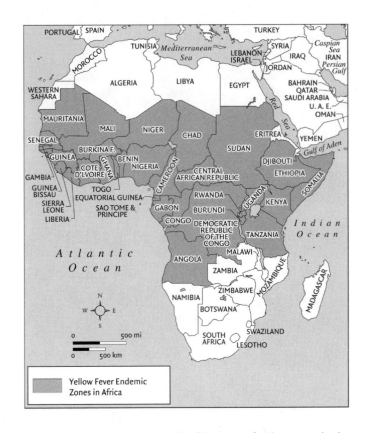

MAP 1 **Distribution of Yellow Fever in Africa.** *Centers for Disease Control and Prevention (www.cdc.gov).*

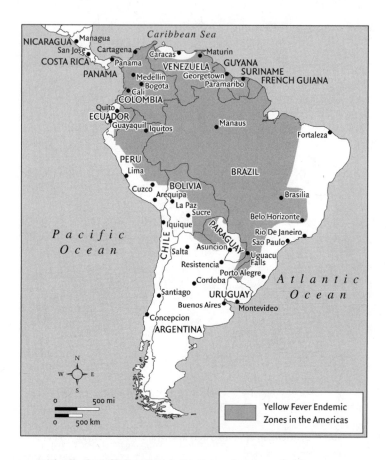

MAP 2 **Distribution of Yellow Fever in South America.** *Centers for Disease Control and Prevention (www.cdc.gov).*

printed on a physician's letterhead, states that you cannot receive yellow fever vaccine for medical reasons. This letter is usually sufficient to get you through customs in countries with yellow fever.

YELLOW FEVER Q & A

Q Wait a minute. You're saying that there is a side effect of receiving the yellow fever vaccine that could kill me—but get the vaccine anyway?

A If you're going to an area with ongoing yellow fever transmission, the risk from vaccination is thought to be less than the risk from yellow fever; so yes, get the vaccine. But suppose you're going only to a city in a country with yellow fever elsewhere—then you might consider getting the exemption letter, particularly if you're elderly, as the elderly are more prone to that rare and horrendous side effect.

MENINGOCOCCAL DISEASE

The only disease aside from yellow fever for which vaccination is sometimes required at international borders is meningococcal disease. Meningococcal meningitis is a life-threatening disease in which the meninges (the lining of the brain) become inflamed. Signs and symptoms are fever, headache, confusion, a stiff neck, and often a rash that looks like a lot of little bruises. Although treatable with common antibiotics if rapidly diagnosed, if untreated it is fatal in over half of cases.

Muslims who make the pilgrimage to Mecca (the Hajj or Umrah) are required to demonstrate current vaccination for meningococcal disease by the Saudi Arabia government. This requirement recently changed, so that the older "bivalent" (providing protection for two subtypes of this illness) vaccine is no longer accepted; the vaccine must be "quadrivalent" (providing protection for four subtypes). All vaccine given in the US is quadrivalent.

Although it is not required, vaccination is strongly recommended for travelers to the African Sahel (the border between the Sahara desert and tropical Africa), an east-to-west stretch of land known as the "meningitis belt" (see map 3). Risk is particularly high during the dry season (December to June). Maps that show the area of transmission of meningococcal meningitis as a single strip across the Sahel are idealized; actually transmission occurs both within that belt and in locations scattered all around it. Travelers visiting any region near the meningitis belt, particularly during the dry months of December through June, should consider this vaccination.

Another situation for which vaccination for this illness is advised is for those living in crowded conditions. In the US this vaccine is advised for all college students living in dorms. Any crowded living situation (e.g., the close quarters of military recruits living in barracks) can increase the risk of transmitting this illness.

There are two forms of the meningococcal vaccine: MPSV4 (Menomune) polysaccharide, which is approved for those above two years of age, and MCV4 conjugate (Menactra), which is approved for those between two and fifty-five years of age.* The conjugate vaccine appears to provide protection for a longer duration than the polysaccharide vaccine; hence for travelers between two and fifty-five years of age, the conjugate is the preferred vaccine.

* Regarding meningococcal vaccine, see the BBC news report at: http://news.bbc.co.uk/1/hi/health/2653759.stm.

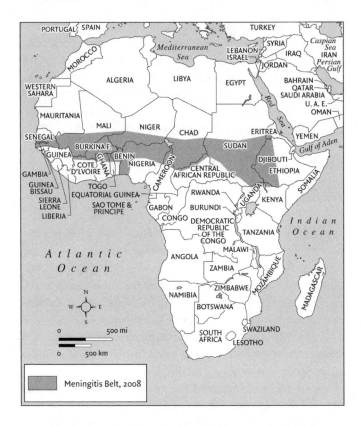

Meningitis Belt, 2008

MAP 3 **Distribution of Meningococcal Meningitis.** *Centers for Disease Control and Prevention (www.cdc.gov).*

The duration of protection from the polysaccharide vaccine is thought to be at least five years in those who receive the vaccine while four years of age or older; revaccination should be considered for those vaccinated while less than four years of age who continue to be at risk. The duration of protection from the conjugate vaccine is longer than that offered by the polysaccharide vaccine but is not known with certainty.

RECOMMENDED VACCINATIONS

TYPHOID FEVER

Typhoid fever, spread by contaminated food and water, is a disease that causes severe gastrointestinal symptoms, including severe abdominal pain, diarrhea that may be bloody (or sometimes constipation), and fever; it can be fatal. It is rare in travelers; risk may be reduced by following the same dietary measures that reduce risk of travelers' diarrhea (see chapter 6).

Typhoid fever vaccine is particularly important for travelers who are going to the developing world for a prolonged duration or are planning particularly rustic travels (e.g., people staying in villages or backpacking). However, travelers should keep in mind that typhoid fever has been contracted by short-stay visitors. Risk is highest in visitors to the Indian subcontinent. Those who choose to receive this vaccine have two options: a single injection or a series of four pills; for most people the pills are preferable. The immunization by injection consists of a single shot. The oral series consists of four pills, taken one every other day on an empty stomach until all four pills are taken. A chief benefit of the pills is that they provide protection for five years, as opposed to only two years for the injection (plus you do not get a shot, always a preferable option). Additionally, the pills are a little cheaper than the vaccine.

JAPANESE ENCEPHALITIS

Japanese encephalitis is caused by a virus that is spread by mosquitoes in rural south and Southeast Asia. Transmission in some countries varies by season: for example, in Vietnam the season of transmission is May to October; in Malaysia transmission is year-round. (A full listing is online at http://www.cdc.gov; click the button to the left that reads "Travelers' health.") Most travelers do not require this vaccine; however, it should be considered by travelers who plan extensive travel in rural south or Southeast Asia, particularly in pig-farming or rice-farming areas. If you're staying in a city, you do not need this vaccine. If you're backpacking, you might.

Only 1 in 200 people who contract Japanese encephalitis will exhibit symptoms, but for that person it's nasty. One-third of people who become symptomatic develop neurological symptoms that fully resolve, one-third develop permanent neurological symptoms (such as paralysis), one-third die.

This vaccine has two major downsides: it is expensive, and it has a high rate of side effects. The three-shot series will run you about $600, and a significant number of recipients will develop bothersome symptoms, including temporary swelling. The vaccine for Japanese encephalitis that is used in the US, which is made by Biken, is no longer being manufactured, and its use is being phased out. (Different vaccines for Japanese encephalitis are used in Asia to immunize children living in endemic areas.) New vaccines are currently being studied in clinical trials, but the timing of future FDA review and licensure of these new vaccines are unknown at this time.

Again, if you're a short-stay tourist staying in towns, you prob-

All Vaccines Are Not Created Equal

When a physician tells you that a vaccine gives you protection for a given disease, you should realize that that protection is usually only partial. For some diseases, including hepatitis A and yellow fever, protection is excellent: less than 1% of people, after receiving these vaccines, will develop illness after being exposed. However, some vaccines offer far less protection. Typhoid fever vaccine (both pills and the shot), for example, offers only about 70% protection, which means that if you administer typhoid fever vaccine to a hundred people, then feed each of them enough typhoid bacteria to cause illness in an unvaccinated person, about thirty people will develop typhoid fever. Seventy percent protection is better than none, so physicians recommend this for adventurous travelers, but there is room for improvement.

ably do not need this vaccine. If you're a wildlife biologist who will be sleeping near rice paddies, the benefits of the protection of the vaccine are probably greater than its risks. This is a vaccine to research, to discuss with your pre-travel provider, to ponder. If the vaccine were cheap and had no side effects, or if the disease were mild, it would be a no-brainer; but as is, it's always a tough call.

RABIES

Rabies is caused by the bite, scratch, or lick of an infected mammal (e.g., dog, cat, bat, rat, monkey). In the developed world, most cases are caused by bites of wild animals; in the developing world, most cases are caused by bites of domesticated animals, e.g., dogs.

As with Japanese encephalitis, the decision whether or not to be vaccinated for rabies can be complex. The problem is that the vaccine is expensive and the disease is extremely rare in travelers; but when it occurs, it is extremely fatal, with 100% of people with rabies dying.

The vaccine series consists of three shots given on days 0, 7, and 21 to 28. Travelers to standard tourist destinations (e.g., beach resorts in Mexico) do not need this vaccine.

Even those who receive this vaccine require additional treatment after potential exposure to rabies: this consists of two shots of rabies vaccine given three days apart. For those who do not receive the pre-exposure series, the post-exposure vaccine series is much more extensive: five shots of rabies vaccine over twenty-eight days, plus a single shot of rabies immune globulin.

If you are bitten by an animal, you should immediately clean the wound with soap and water; this will kill a significant amount of the rabies virus should it be present (although not so much that

Who Should Get Pre-Exposure Rabies Vaccine

+ Veterinarians, wildlife biologists
+ Backpackers
+ People who travel to remote, isolated areas
+ Travelers planning prolonged time abroad

you want to forgo "post-exposure prophylaxis"—injections after the bite). Whether or not you've had the pre-exposure series of rabies vaccine, you want to initiate post-exposure vaccine as soon as possible after an exposure, preferably within one to two days.

Note: None of the rabies shots—neither the series prior to exposure nor the ones after exposure—is into the abdomen or particularly painful. They are simply standard shots into your upper arm. The painful injections into the abdomen haven't been given for decades.

TWO NONRECOMMENDATIONS

CHOLERA

Cholera, a diarrheal illness causing life-threatening dehydration, is phenomenally rare in tourists. Cholera vaccine is not available in the US and is not recommended for any traveler, regardless of destination or planned activities. An oral cholera vaccine is available in Western Europe, Asia, and Canada (see pp. 149–50).

SMALLPOX

Smallpox has been eradicated. The last naturally occurring case occurred in Somalia in 1977. There is no need for smallpox vaccine for any traveler.

VACCINE INTERACTIONS

Live vaccines should be given either on the same day or separated by at least twenty-eight days.

Oral typhoid vaccine is live and hence can be inactivated by some antibiotics and antimalarials, including doxycycline and

Malarone. Travelers should wait at least two weeks after finishing the four capsules of oral typhoid vaccine before taking doxycycline, Malarone, or other drugs that could interfere with the typhoid vaccine. The antimalarials mefloquine (Lariam) and chloroquine (Aralen) do not decrease the effectiveness of oral typhoid vaccine.

There is no interaction between the typhoid vaccine by injection, which is a killed vaccine, and oral medications.

A full list of vaccine interactions and contraindications is available at the CDC site, at: http://www.cdc.gov/nip/recs.contraindications.htm.

VFRs: A High-Risk Group

One group of international travelers who are at particularly high risk for infectious diseases when they travel from the developed to the developing world are "VFRs"—"visiting friends and relatives": those who have immigrated to a developed country such as the US or Western Europe, then return to their home in the developing world. There are many possible explanations for this increased risk; one is that VFRs may pooh-pooh the dangers of their native land and fail to see a pre-travel provider. VFRs are by no means exempt from the dictum that all international travelers to the developing world should see a pre-travel provider; indeed, given that many VFRs travel rurally and for long durations, they may benefit from pre-travel care even more than the average traveler.

VACCINE MYTHS

"Vaccines can cause autism in children."

There is no evidence that links vaccines to autism or any other developmental or psychiatric illness. British researchers A. J. Wakefield and colleagues did publish one paper that suggested a link between measles-mumps-rubella (MMR) vaccine and autism. No one has been able to replicate their findings, which is doctor talk for something was funny about their research. It is difficult to prove a negative, but among the evidence that autism and vaccines are not linked:

+ The MMR vaccine was introduced in England in 1988; there was no increase in autism following this introduction.
+ Autism is not more common in children who have been immunized with MMR than in those who have not.
+ Autism diagnoses do not cluster about the time of MMR vaccine administration.

"I don't want to overwhelm my body's immune system by getting too many vaccines at once."

Your body can develop antibodies to hundreds of thousands, if not millions, of different germs. Receiving vaccines for several diseases at once does not overwhelm your body, or cause the vaccines to work less well.

"Chickenpox is always a mild illness, so why get vaccinated?"

Prior to the introduction of chickenpox vaccine in the mid-1990s, approximately 11,000 people were hospitalized and 100 people died each year in the US from this illness. It's mild in many kids, but some children and most adults with chickenpox are miserable for weeks; some become critically ill.

"I'm late in getting the second or third shot in a series, so I have to start over."

With the exception of oral typhoid vaccine, vaccines can be given late with no loss in protection once the series is completed. For example, suppose you had the first hepatitis A shot three years ago. (The usual schedule is to have two shots six to twelve months apart.) A single hepatitis A shot will provide protection for six to twelve months; protection will then wane unless the second shot is given. After the second shot is given, however, long-term immunity is just as solid as if the shots had been given exactly on schedule. In other words, once the series is complete, there is no penalty for some shots being given late.

A CAVEAT

Pregnant women, and people who are immunosuppressed, should not receive live vaccines, which include: measles, mumps, rubella, oral typhoid, oral polio, intranasal flu, yellow fever, BCG (for tuberculosis), and varicella (chickenpox). Note: Oral polio vaccine is no longer given in the US. BCG is administered to children in most of the world but not in the US.

HOW TO PRIORITIZE, OR, WHAT TO DO WHEN THE TRAVEL PROVIDER RECOMMENDS MORE VACCINES THAN YOU CAN AFFORD

Vaccines aren't cheap and it's quite possible that your pre-travel provider will recommend more vaccines than you can afford. It is reasonable to ask your provider to rank these for you, in order of most-to-least beneficial.

SCENARIO #1

Suppose you are going to Mexico and your pre-travel provider, after reviewing your generally complete vaccine record (which, incidentally, you should always take with you when visiting your pre-travel clinic if possible), advises that you get vaccines for hepatitis A, typhoid, and rabies. You have only $70 allotted for vaccines. What to do?

Well, the three-shot rabies series is about $700, so that's right out. Ask the provider (realizing that it's fully permissible and appropriate to talk with physicians and other medical personnel about cost) which is more important, and he or she will probably say: hepatitis A. (Both hepatitis A and typhoid are serious illnesses, but hepatitis A is *much* more common.)

SCENARIO #2

You're taking a whole year to travel around the world. You've allotted $300 for vaccines. Your travel clinic provider advises seven vaccines, which cost over $1,000. Your provider then, at your request, prioritizes these.

You decide to get the first five on the list, which are hepatitis A, tetanus-diphtheria, yellow fever, typhoid fever (oral), and influenza; you pass on rabies and Japanese encephalitis. (You probably don't need the vaccine for Japanese encephalitis as you're not spending time in rural Southeast Asia, and you promise that if you're bitten, scratched, or otherwise exposed to mammal spit, you'll see a medical provider ASAP [preferably within 24 hours] for the postexposure rabies vaccine series.)

SCENARIO #3

You plan to visit Thailand and Vietnam. Your pre-travel provider advises yellow fever vaccine.

Your response: Get a new pre-travel provider. There is no yellow fever anywhere in Asia.

SCENARIO #4

You are a little allergic to eggs: you can eat one with no problems, but if you eat two or more you develop nausea and hives. Your travel provider advises that you get one or more of the vaccines that contain eggs (yellow fever, influenza [by injection, not intranasal], mumps, measles).

Your response: Get the vaccine(s) as advised. The amount of egg in vaccines is minuscule; if you can eat one egg without ill effects, you're good to get the vaccine.

SCENARIO #5

You're *really* allergic to eggs. If you eat even a tiny bit you swell up or worse.

Your response: See an allergist, who can skin test you with the vaccine. Typically they will dilute the vaccine with water, then inject a little under your skin. If a hive appears, then you do not get the vaccine. If it's a required vaccine, such as yellow fever, then have either the allergist or your pre-travel provider write a note on physician's letterhead stating that you are exempt for medical reasons; these are almost always accepted at international borders.

VACCINE Q & A

Q What if I only have time to receive a portion of a vaccine
series prior to my departure?

A In general, if you only receive a portion of a vaccine series
you will have some protection, but not as much as if you had
received the entire series. An exception is hepatitis A: after one
dose of hepatitis A, you are fully protected for six to twelve
months.

3 Malaria

THE BOTTOM LINE

+ Malaria is a life-threatening disease. It remains a threat throughout the tropics; each year it kills over a million people, most of them children in Africa.

+ The two key components of avoiding malaria are "personal protection measures" (i.e., avoiding mosquito bites) and taking a preventative medication.

Malaria is a phenomenally unpleasant disease. Those with malaria develop extremely high fevers, they perspire to the extent that they are lying in puddles of sweat, and they shake as though stuck to an electric fence. Every year malaria kills over a million people. While I am a proponent of returning home with travel stories, no tale is worth the suffering that malaria causes. Plus, if you die, it will not be you but your next of kin who will be telling the story, which is, from your point of view, a suboptimal situation.

A key aspect of malaria is that it is spread by mosquitoes; if you're not bitten by a mosquito, your risk of contracting malaria plummets. Hence the first topic to discuss is not drugs to prevent malaria, but strategies by which to avoid bug bites.

INSECT AVOIDANCE MEASURES

Minimizing mosquito bites is fully as important as taking a proper medication; some authorities state that it's more important.

DEET TO EXPOSED SKIN

By far the best insect repellent is DEET. Frankly, I wish it weren't so. DEET has a petrochemical smell and, in high concentrations, dissolves plastic. However, in terms of both its power to repel mosquitoes and its very minimal side effect profile, nothing approaches it. In June 2006, *Consumer Reports* published the results of its independent testing of eighteen insect repellents. The top seven brands were all DEET products.

Doctors do not talk like ordinary people. When a physician states, "DEET has a favorable risk-to-benefit ratio," what they mean is: "DEET is good. It does what you want it to and it doesn't do much of what you don't want it to." In addition to repelling mosquitoes, DEET also repels ticks, fleas, chiggers, biting flies, and midges. Over 20,000 compounds have been tested as potential insect repellents over the past forty years; none has been superior to DEET.

DEET should only be applied to *exposed* skin, not beneath clothes, not onto clothes. Additionally, DEET should be used in moderation or not at all on damaged (e.g., by abrasion or sunburn) skin. Damaged skin can allow increased absorption of DEET, which can potentially lead to a higher risk of toxicity.

DEET can irritate the skin and, if absorbed in large amounts, can cause neurological symptoms, but these effects are rare.

Whereas some backpacking supply businesses market preparations of 100% DEET, the recommended concentration is in the range of 20 to 35%; this provides all the protection of the higher concentrations, with less risk of skin irritation.

Overall, DEET is wonderful: bugs hate it, and almost no one gets irritated skin or other side effects from it. And it's cheap. In medical practice you rarely find this combination of powerful efficacy, minimal side effects, and affordability.

DEET is safe for use during pregnancy.

PERMETHRIN TO CLOTHES

Similarly, permethrin is great stuff. A synthetic chemical related to pyrethrum, found in the chrysanthemum, permethrin is cheap and doesn't leave a smell. Bugs touch it and they drop dead.

Unlike DEET, permethrin is applied to your clothes. It comes in two forms: as a solution that you dip your clothes into, or as a liquid in a spray pump bottle. You should put permethrin on all your clothes: pants, shirt, socks, hat, bandana. You can even put it on delicate synthetics such as rayon and nylon. Do not

Permethrin Testimonial

In 2001 I volunteered at a remote jungle clinic in the Peruvian Amazon, about fifty miles downriver from Iquitos. While I've always used DEET, this was my first trip during which I used permethrin, and I found that I was bitten significantly less than any prior to trip to buggy environs.

wear your clothes as you apply permethrin, and apply it in a well-ventilated area. One application will give benefit for at least two weeks, despite laundering your clothes.

In a study in Alaska, subjects who applied DEET to their exposed skin and wore permethrin-treated clothes saw over a 99.9% reduction in bug bites; they were bitten once per hour. Subjects in another group, who used neither DEET nor permethrin, were bitten by insects an average of 1,188 times per hour, which tells us:

+ the combination of DEET and permethrin make a formidable barrier to insects, and
+ never volunteer for a study on insect repellents.

BEDNET

Sleeping under a bednet—ideally one treated with permethrin— will markedly reduce your bites by insects, including mosquitoes. Additionally, it will keep all nocturnal creepy-crawlies off you. There is nothing so disconcerting as waking up at night in the jungle as something scampers across your face.

CLOTHING

Wearing long pants and long-sleeved shirts will reduce your risk of insect-transmitted diseases, including malaria. This is a standard recommendation, and it does help, but this is the one bit of bug avoidance advice that I personally have trouble with. Buggy regions tend to be hot and muggy; long pants and sleeves will make you sweat all the more.

The mosquitoes that transmit malaria (genus *Anopheles*) bite at night; thus minimizing your time outdoors at night will reduce your risk of *Anopheles* mosquito bites. Every species of *Anopheles* mosquito has its specific feeding patterns. *Anopheles gambiae*, the principal vector of malaria in Africa, bites late at night; *Anopheles darlingi*, an important vector in the Amazon Basin of South America, feeds earlier in the evening. Hence the use of permethrin-impregnated bed nets is particularly important in areas with malaria in Africa, and personal protection measures (DEET to exposed skin, permethrin to clothes, etc.) are particularly important in areas with malaria in the Amazon Basin, although both strategies should be employed in both areas.

HABITAT AVOIDANCE

Insects tend to like stagnant water. If you're camping, set up your tent in a high, dry, open area, away from rivers and other bodies of water.

INSECT AVOIDANCE MEASURES Q & A

Q DEET stinks. And it dissolves plastic! What is it doing to my chromosomes?

A DEET was put on the market in 1957; currently, worldwide, over 200 million people use DEET every year. If it did something funky to our chromosomes, we'd probably know about it by now.

Q **What about herbal repellents?**

A While a few of these have been shown to have some ability to repel some insects, none of them approach the bug-repelling power of DEET. Citronella, verbena, basil, and garlic have been reported to have short-term (under two hours) repellent properties.

Q **So all right-minded people agree that DEET is best?**

A No. The favorite insect repellent of Scott Carroll, an evolutionary biologist and entomologist at the University of California, Davis, is Avon Skin So Soft Plus IR3535 20%. He's also keen on the Repel brand of oil of lemon eucalyptus.

Q **What about ultrasound devices? I've seen ads that say these gizmos imitate the sounds of bats or dragonflies and frighten the mosquitoes away. And what about electronic buzzers, and vitamin B1 (thiamine)?**

A They don't work.

Q **Ernest Hemingway wrote that when he was hunting in Africa, tobacco smoke would keep the bugs away. Does that work?**

A Maybe it was his smell that kept the bugs away. Tobacco smoke doesn't keep bugs away. (I performed a small experiment in eastern Washington State. While camping by a lake, I sat outside at dusk and smoked several clove cigarettes. Not only did I develop nausea [I don't smoke], but I was bitten by mosquitoes on every square inch of exposed skin.) Additionally, as Hemingway noted, his technique only works if you're downwind from the game; if you're upwind the game will smell you. Thus if you're utilizing the Hemingway technique and the wind changes, you may experience a reversal of the hunter-prey relationship that you initially envisaged.

ANTIMALARIALS

The second key component of malaria avoidance is taking an appropriate antimalarial drug. Every year approximately 1,000 US citizens develop malaria; almost 100% of these people were not taking a preventative medicine or were taking an inappropriate drug.

It is helpful to think of malaria as falling into one of two categories: chloroquine-sensitive and chloroquine-resistant.

CHLOROQUINE-SENSITIVE MALARIA

Chloroquine (trade name in the US: Aralen; trade names outside the US include Resorchin, Avloclor, and Nivaquine) remains effective in preventing malaria in only a handful of the approximately 100 countries with malaria.

Chloroquine-Sensitive Countries

+ Mexico
+ Central America: Belize, Costa Rica, El Salvador, Guatemala, Honduras, Nicaragua, and Panama to the west of the Panama Canal
+ The Island of Hispaniola (the Dominican Republic and Haiti)
+ South America: northern Argentina, Paraguay

- A few of the newly independent states of the former Soviet Union: Azerbaijan, Georgia, Kyrgyzstan, Turkmenistan, Uzbekistan, Armenia
- Elsewhere: Iraq, North Korea, South Korea, Mauritius, Syria, Turkey

Note: Chloroquine-sensitive malaria is also present in North Africa (Algeria, Egypt, Morocco, western Sahara), but the areas with malaria are quite small, and the CDC does not recommend that travelers to these countries take prophylactic medication.

For most travelers to chloroquine-sensitive areas, I prescribe not chloroquine but hydroxychloroquine (Plaquenil), a near-identical drug. I do this because Plaquenil, in the US, costs one-fifth of what chloroquine does. If you're buying it outside the US, you will not face the same pricing differential, so either one is fine.

Chloroquine schedule: This drug is taken once/week. You start one week before entry into the area with malaria, take it once/week while there, and—this last bit is important—you take it for four weeks after you exit the malaria area. Adult dose: 500 mg/week.

Plaquenil schedule: This drug is taken once/week. You start one week before entry into the area with malaria, you take it once/week while there, and—this last bit is important—you take it for four weeks after you exit the malaria area. Adult dose: 400 mg/week.

Chloroquine and Plaquenil side effects: Most people who take these drugs have no side effects. Rare side effects include rash, stomach upset, and mood changes. Chloroquine may exacerbate psoriasis.

In all countries with malaria other than those listed above, malaria is resistant to chloroquine. The CDC recommends that you take one of three drugs while in areas with chloroquine-resistant malaria. All have pros and cons; your choice will depend on the duration of your stay, your pocketbook, and minimizing your chance of side effects.

Doxycycline

Doxycycline is an underutilized and underappreciated drug for the prevention of chloroquine-resistant malaria. It's dirt cheap—about sixteen to eighteen cents/pill, and most people have no side effects. It doesn't receive the advertising budget of Malarone, because it is available in generic form and hence profits to pharmaceutics companies are meager, but particularly for long-stay travelers or those on a tight budget, it's often the best choice.

Doxycycline schedule: This drug is taken once/day. You begin one day prior to arrival in the malaria area, you continue taking it once/day while there, and you take it for twenty-eight days after leaving the malaria area. Adult dose: 100 mg once/day.

You should not take doxycycline if you are under eight years of age, pregnant, or a sexually active woman of childbearing years and not using birth control.

The most common possible side effects of doxycycline are stomach upset and photosensitivity (light sensitivity). A small number of people who take doxycycline will find that the sun causes a rash. This side effect used to be thought to be fairly common; recent studies show that less than 1% of people who take doxycycline develop this reaction. (One reason that people who take doxycycline for malaria prevention see a low rate of photosensitivity is that they take only 100 mg/day, which is half the dose taken for an infection such as urethritis.) Given the low cost of doxycycline, consider asking your pre-travel provider to write for a few—say three—extra pills. Prior to your trip, take a pill once/day for three days and either get some natural sun or spend ten minutes in a tanning parlor. If nothing untoward happens to your skin, doxycycline is unlikely to make you sun sensitive when you take it for a longer duration.

Doxycycline also increases the likelihood of vaginal yeast infections. A potential side effect of doxycycline is esophageal ulceration. Doxycycline should not be swallowed "dry," but with a generous volume of a liquid. If this pill gets stuck part way down your esophagus, it can cause an esophageal ulceration, which is a serious complication, and will necessitate ending your trip and flying to the developed world for treatment.

A benefit of taking doxycycline for malaria is that if you are engaged in a freshwater sport such as kayaking, the doxycycline will simultaneously prevent you from getting leptospirosis, a disease that is not uncommonly spread by contact with fresh water in the developing world (see section on leptospirosis in chapter 5).

Malarone (atovaquone/proguanil)

Released onto the US drug market in 2000, Malarone is the newest of the three drugs recommended by the CDC for prevention of chloroquine-resistant malaria. Malarone, a combination of two drugs, atovaquone and proguanil, is taken daily. It has the lowest risk of side effects of the three options in chloroquine-resistant areas; unfortunately, it's also by far the priciest of the three.

Schedule: Malarone is taken once/day. Start one day before arriving in the malaria area, take once/day while there, and continue taking it once/day for seven days after leaving the malaria area. (This is more convenient than taking doxycycline or mefloquine, each of which is taken for four weeks after leaving the malaria area [doxycycline daily, mefloquine weekly].) For adults, Malarone comes as a fixed combination tablet of 250 mg atovaquone and 100 mg proguanil.

Malarone side effects: Malarone's claim to fame is its favorable side effect profile. You can get a rash, or stomach upset, or even psychiatric side effects from Malarone, but these are rare. Most people have no side effects at all.

Mefloquine (Lariam)

If this drug were a Top-40 pop song, it would be said to be bubbling under: still on the charts, but drifting downward. It remains a good drug for many people, but due to a significant rate of neurological and psychiatric side effects, its popularity is on the wane.

Mefloquine schedule: A single 250 milligram tablet is taken by adults once/week. Start one week before arriving at the malaria area, take it once/week while there, and continue for four weeks after leaving the malaria area. The cost is intermediate between doxycycline and Malarone: about five dollars/pill.

Potential side effects of mefloquine include: vivid dreams or nightmares, anxiety, depression, and (rarely) psychosis. And of course it carries risk for those side effects which most drugs have: rash and GI upset.

Who Should Avoid Mefloquine?

+ Anyone who has ever had any sort of mood disorder, such as depression or anxiety, should not take mefloquine, as those people have an increased risk of neuropsychiatric side effects, including depression and anxiety. Even if you're fine now, but had an episode of depression a while back—stay away from mefloquine.

+ Anyone with a history of cardiac conduction defects ("heart block") should avoid this drug.
+ Anyone with any history of seizures (aside from uncomplicated febrile seizures as a child) should stay away from mefloquine, as it "lowers the seizure threshold"—that is, makes seizure more likely.
+ Anyone who has had an adverse reaction to mefloquine in the past.
+ Anyone who doesn't want to take it.

Note: If you're traveling with small children, store your antimalarial medication on a high shelf, in a childproof container. Consuming even a small number of pills of antimalarial medication can cause severe illness or death in children.

ANTIMALARIA DRUGS Q & A

Q With all those side effects, should anyone take mefloquine?

A Most people who take mefloquine have no side effects at all. If you've taken it before and done well on it, the odds that it'll do something nasty are quite low, and it would be reasonable to try it again. (I take mefloquine when I'm in areas with chloroquine-resistant malaria and I've never had any side effects. My friends have made a number of small remarks as to why I don't notice its crazy-making side effects.)

Q After what I've heard about mefloquine, there is no way I'm taking it. Should I just avoid malaria drugs altogether?

A No. There are two other perfectly good drugs—doxycycline and

Malarone—for the prevention of chloroquine-resistant malaria. Take one of those two.

Q Every time I take mefloquine, I get vivid dreams. I kind of like them. Should I stop taking mefloquine?

A No. Some people enjoy the vivid dreams they have while taking mefloquine, and refer to the night after the day on which they take the mefloquine, when dreams tend to be particularly vivid, as "movie night." As long as you're not developing side effects that you do not like, such as nightmares or anxiety, there is no problem in continuing to take the mefloquine.

Q I'm going to be in an area with chloroquine-resistant malaria for a long time—two years. I'm taking doxycycline because it's the cheapest. Can I really take it for two years? Should I take a break now and then?

A Yes, you could and should take it for two years. In the US dermatologists routinely give adolescents doxycycline (or a closely related drug, minocycline) for acne for several years, and most develop no side effects. And no, taking a break is a very bad idea. Malaria can be a life-threatening illness, and it does your body no good to take the occasional "holiday" from the drug.

When the cumulative dose of chloroquine (Aralen) or hydroxy-chloroquine (Plaquenil) exceeds 100 g (which is usually reached in adults after five to six years of continuous use), there is risk of retinal toxicity. Those who take chloroquine or hydroxychloroquine for over five years should have an ophthalmologic examination every six months, and change to another antimalarial medication should there be any signs of retinal damage.

Q We're going to an area with malaria for our honeymoon. Which of these drugs is least risky for me to get pregnant on?

A None of these has been proven safe in pregnancy. There are a small number of drugs, such as acetaminophen (Tylenol) and penicillin, that have been shown to be safe at any stage of pregnancy. And there are a small number of drugs that have been shown to be harmful during pregnancy, such as, to give an extreme example, thalidomide. Most drugs fall into a middle ground: no deleterious effect on the fetus has been identified, but no studies have been done, and we do not really know.

Doxycycline should never be taken during pregnancy as it can cause a baby's teeth to be stained yellow-brown after birth. Although some authorities state that mefloquine, Malarone, and chloroquine are safe to use during pregnancy, large studies have not been performed, and ideally, pregnant women should postpone travel to areas with malaria. If travel to an area with malaria is essential, the risk from these drugs may indeed be lower than that from malaria, particularly in someone visiting an area with intense transmission of malaria, such as sub-Saharan Africa.

Q So should I take nothing for malaria prevention at all while there?

A No! Malaria is a life-threatening illness, and furthermore, pregnant women and their fetuses do particularly poorly when they get malaria. You should use birth control while in the malaria area; then, if you want to attempt pregnancy, do not stop using the birth control until you have been off the malaria medications for a month.

Q But we really want to try to get pregnant on our honeymoon, and our hearts are set on a tropical destination.

A No problem. Plenty of tropical islands—Hawaii, the Bahamas, Fiji, and French Polynesia including Tahiti, among others—are free of malaria. Consider going to one of those.

Q I've heard that medications are much cheaper abroad than in the US. Is there a problem with just buying the malaria medication once I arrive?

A Potentially, yes. Quality control of pharmaceuticals in the developing world is spotty, and a significant number of placebo pills (pills with sugar or some other chemical without pharmacological action) are sold in pharmacies. One study showed that as many as one pill in three sold in developing world pharmacies, among more expensive drugs, was adulterated, post-dated, or bogus. Another recent study found that at least twelve counterfeit preparations of artesunate, a medication used to treat malaria, were on the market in Southeast Asia. Given that malaria is a life-threatening illness, the best course is to buy the drugs in the developed world.

Q I'm taking over 100 doxycycline tablets with me for a prolonged stay. Am I going to have trouble at customs?

A As long as you keep the pills in the labeled container provided at the pharmacy, almost certainly not. Do not put the pills into an envelope, plastic bag, or other informal container. Loose, unlabeled pills, particularly in large volumes, can draw unwelcome scrutiny at customs.

Q You're saying that the dosing schedule for each drug includes taking it for some time after I leave the malaria area?

A Yes. Chloroquine, Plaquenil, mefloquine, and doxycycline are taken for four weeks after exiting the malaria area; Malarone is taken for one week after exiting the malaria area. The reason ties into the life cycle of the malaria parasite. Suppose you are taking an appropriate drug for malaria prevention, and you are bitten by a mosquito that is transmitting malaria. The mosquito injects the malaria parasite (a one-celled protozoan organism of the genus *Plasmodium*) into your bloodstream—the drug doesn't stop that. The malaria parasite rapidly travels to your liver—the drug doesn't stop that. The malaria parasite multiplies in your liver—the drug doesn't stop that (except Malarone, which does kill the liver stage of the parasite).

Q Wait a minute. The parasite multiplies in my liver even if I'm taking the right drug? Don't I feel sick at this point?

A No. You feel fine. Then the malaria parasite leaves your liver and starts to multiply in your bloodstream. This is when you would start to feel sick if you were not taking an antimalarial. And this is when the drug works. The malaria parasite, after it exits your liver, is prevented from multiplying. You continue to feel fine, and are not aware that it's been in your liver or elsewhere.

Q I was born and raised in an area with year-round malaria transmission. I'm immune, right?

A It is true that those who survive childhood in areas with year-round malaria transmission will develop "semi-immunity." Semi-immunity reduces the symptoms of malaria. Infection in a nonimmune person causes misery for weeks or is fatal; malaria infection in those with semi-immunity is much milder, akin to a bad cold. But a key point regarding semi-immunity to malaria is that if a person with semi-immunity leaves the malaria area for even a year or two, that partial protection disappears and malaria is again a life-threatening infection. There are numerous accounts of people born and raised in equatorial Africa who then attend school in the UK or US, only to be killed by their first bout of malaria when they return to their nation of birth.

Q What is "terminal prophylaxis"?

A Infection with two of the four types of malaria, P. vivax and P. ovale, can lead to relapses years after the initial exposure. For travelers who have had prolonged exposure in malaria-endemic areas (such as Peace Corps volunteers or missionaries), terminal prophylaxis, also known as presumptive anti-relapse therapy, or "the chaser," is sometimes advised to reduce the risk of relapse. This entails taking the drug primaquine for fourteen days (30 mg of base once/day for adults). **Important:** Anyone who plans on taking primaquine must first be screened for G6PD-deficiency, an enzyme deficiency that is particularly common among those of African, Middle Eastern, and Southeast Asian descent. Regardless of race, all people must be screened for this condition prior to taking primaquine. People with G6PD deficiency who take primaquine can develop life-threatening hemolysis (bursting of red blood cells). Only people with a normal G6PD level can take primaquine.

For those who take chloroquine, Plaquenil, doxycycline, or mefloquine for malaria prophylaxis, the fourteen days of primaquine can be taken during the final two weeks of the four weeks of the postexposure prophylaxis, or immediately after. For those who take Malarone (atovaquone/proguanil), the fourteen days of primaquine can be taken for the seven days of postexposure prophylaxis and for one week thereafter, or for the two weeks immediately following the one week of postexposure prophylaxis.

THE CARRY-ALONG STRATEGY, A.K.A. PRESUMPTIVE SELF-TREATMENT OF MALARIA, A.K.A. STAND-BY EMERGENCY SELF-TREATMENT (SBET)

This is controversial. I have strong opinions, which I will share. The rationale for carry-along drugs for malaria goes something like this: The drugs have side effects, and most people do not get malaria. Isn't it wiser to take nothing beforehand, then take a curative medication if malaria occurs?

In a word, no. The strongest argument against the carry-along strategy is that without a medical laboratory and a trained technician, you cannot tell if you have malaria or not. Suppose you're in the jungles of Papua New Guinea and you develop high fevers and achy joints. Do you have malaria? Maybe. Do you have dengue fever? Maybe. Do you have influenza? Maybe. Do you have something else? Maybe. You cannot tell if someone has malaria or not by the symptoms. Even a physician who specializes in tropical medicine, after a detailed history and a full physical exam, cannot tell if someone does or does not have malaria without laboratory tests.

Swiss and German studies showed that travelers overused presumptive self-treatment for malaria between four fold and ten fold. Putting this differently, of those travelers who took the self-treatment medicine for presumed malaria, only 10 to 25% actually had malaria. In November 2006 Dr. Lin Chen and colleagues published an excellent overview of prevention of malaria in long-term travelers in the *Journal of the American Medical Association* in which they concluded, "Self-diagnosis of malaria is unlikely to be correct."

So the whole concept of "when I get malaria I'll just do such-and-so" is flawed because when you get a fever and chills, you don't know whether or not you have malaria. Some illnesses that cause fever are minor; some are life-threatening. Additionally, the treatment regimens themselves have high rates of side effects, and you hate to expose yourself to those potential adverse effects if you may not have malaria. However, the carry-along strategy continues to be utilized by some travelers, and you will no doubt come across travelers who will tell you that you're a fool to take a poisonous medication for your entire stay in a malaria area. As I say, it remains controversial.

The one situation for which you might consider the carry-along strategy would be if you are extremely remote geographically, that is, if it would take you a long time to reach medical care should you fall ill. Always consult with your pre-travel provider should this be your plan.

Currently there are several commercial kits with which you prick yourself with a needle, put a drop of blood onto a card, and add various reagents; a particular color change indicates that you have malaria. Currently these tests are cumbersome and relatively inaccurate. At some time in the future, when these malaria diagnostic kits are as simple and accurate as home pregnancy tests, self-treatment will be an option, but we're not there yet.

MALARIA Q & A

Q Is malaria in tourists rare?

A No. Every year approximately 30,000 residents of industrialized nations who visit the developing world contract malaria. The

Will Mefloquine Make Me Crazy?

This is one of the most controversial topics within travel medicine. There are ongoing class-action lawsuits in the United Kingdom regarding alleged permanent damage to folks' psyches caused by mefloquine. There are a number of people who say this is Satan's medicine, that only a dunce would take it.

What is true is that mefloquine causes side effects, including changes of mood, in a proportion of people who take it. It can cause anxiety, or depression, or nightmares; these symptoms resolve after the drug is stopped. And very rarely—perhaps in one person in ten thousand—it can cause outright psychosis, which abates when the drug is stopped.

On the one hand, malaria is a life-threatening illness, and the risk-benefit ratio for mefloquine is favorable when compared to risks and benefits of other drugs that we commonly use. On the other hand, there are two other drugs, Malarone and doxycycline, which have a lower rate of neuropsychiatric side effects, that protect equally well against chloroquine-resistant malaria.

The bottom line is that if you have taken mefloquine before and done well, you'll probably do well on it in the future. If you've never taken it, one of the other two—doxycycline or Malarone—should probably be your first choice.

great majority of them were taking the wrong medication for the prevention of malaria or no medication at all.

Q Are there any other preventative measures that long-term visitors can undertake?

A Putting screens on windows and eliminating pools of standing water in which mosquitoes can breed (e.g., flowerpots) in the vicinity of your dwelling will reduce risk.

Q Should I take a preventative medication only during the rainy season?

A While it's true that some countries, e.g., Botswana and Namibia, have both high- and low-transmission seasons, risk persists during the low-transmission season. Additionally, unusual weather patterns can vary the usual pattern. As a general rule, travelers should not discontinue their preventative antimalarial medication during the "off-season."

Q I've heard that qinghaosu from China is a good antimalarial. Can I use that for malaria prevention?

A Qinghaosu (more commonly known in the Western world as artemisinin) is in fact the most powerful antimalarial drug known to man. Derived from the shrub *Artemisia annua*, qinghaosu has been used by Chinese herbalists to treat malaria and other illnesses for over a thousand years. Due to the poor bioavailability of artemisinin, semi-synthetic derivatives have been developed, including artemether and artesunate. However, the half-life of these drugs (the duration they remain in your bloodstream) is too brief to work as effective preventative medications; they are only employed for the treatment of malaria. They are best taken in combination with another drug, such as lumefantrine. See information at WHO web site (http://www.who.org) on artemisinin-based combination therapy (ACT).

Q I take minocycline (or doxycycline) daily for acne (or another condition). I'm going to an area for which an antimalarial is advised. What should I do?

A If you're on doxycycline 100 mg once/day, stay on it. If you're on minocycline, change to doxycycline 100 mg once/day, for the duration advised for malaria (start one day before arrival, once/day during your time there, and once/day for twenty-eight days after leaving), then switch back to minocycline. Doxycycline works for both chloroquine-sensitive and chloroquine-resistant areas.

Q Do any other antibiotics protect against malaria?

A Some offer partial protection, but none offers sufficient protection, other than those mentioned above.

Q Can't I just be vaccinated for malaria?

A An effective vaccine for malaria does not yet exist. Although promising reports on new malaria vaccines are published regularly, it will probably be many years until an effective vaccine hits the market.

4 Urban Medicine

THREATS TO HEALTH OF TRAVELERS TO CITIES

~~~~~~

THE BOTTOM LINE

+ Most deaths of young, fit travelers are due to road traffic accidents.

+ Seat belts are good.

+ Don't ride in the back of a truck or on the roof of a bus.

+ Stay off the roads at night.

+ Don't ride mopeds or motorcycles.

+ If you have sex with a new partner, using condoms is smart. Not using condoms is dumb.

~~~~~~

Even if your ultimate destination is rural and remote, you almost always must transit through a big city en route. Most travelers to the game parks of East Africa fly into Nairobi, population 2.5 million; most travelers to the beaches of southern Thailand fly into Bangkok, population 6 million; most travelers set on trekking to Machu Picchu in Peru fly into Lima, population 8 million. Surviving the megacity is requisite for arriving at your final and rustic destination.

And I would not try to dissuade you from visiting developing world big cities. Poor big cities are wonderful and terrible at the same time; they contain the best and the worst of humanity. But—and this is my key point—preparation and particular strategies can minimize your chance of something untoward occurring while in the metropolis.

When most people think about threats to health of international travelers, their first thought is infectious disease: malaria, yellow fever, cholera. However, studies that look at the causes of death of those who foray from affluent countries to the developing world consistently show that infectious diseases—all infectious diseases, including pneumonia, malaria, yellow fever, cholera, kidney infections, skin infections—account for only about 1% of deaths. About half the deaths are due to heart attacks and strokes; these occur primarily in the elderly. So what is the most common cause of death in young healthy travelers?

Simple: road traffic accidents, including car crashes, motorcycle crashes, and bus crashes. Road traffic accidents are the number one cause of demise of nonelderly international travelers. Even a 10% reduction in deaths in international travelers due to motor vehicle crashes would save more lives than would total elimination of deaths in international travelers from all infectious diseases.

ROAD TRAFFIC ACCIDENTS

The unfortunate truth is that road traffic accidents are much, much more common in the developing world. Some statistics: The rate of fatalities per 100 million miles driven in the US is 1.1; this is similar to rates in Western Europe. The rates in Sri Lanka

Priorities

Suppose that you were to see a pre-travel provider for a one-hour counseling session prior to your vacation to a developing nation, and further suppose that that provider spent time on various topics in direct proportion to that topic's likelihood of causing your death during your travels. In this scenario, your pre-travel provider would spend thirty minutes on mundane topics such as cholesterol, exercise, weight, smoking, and blood pressure, in an effort to reduce your risk of heart attack and stroke. Then you would get about fifteen minutes on the benefits of seat belts and helmets, including a host of caveats: Do not ride on the roof of a bus, even if you're told the view is terrific. Do not ride in the back of an open truck. Do not rent a motorcycle or moped. Avoid driving at night. You would then hear about fourteen minutes regarding other causes of premature demise, including drowning, homicide, falls from heights. And finally, for thirty-six seconds, you would hear about all infectious diseases: influenza, pneumonia, hepatitis A, B, and C, malaria, typhoid fever, HIV, etc. In fact, most pre-travel providers spend the bulk of their time on infectious diseases, but as you can infer, I think that that allotment of time is suboptimal. No one sees a pre-travel provider to hear about seat belts and not riding in the backs of open trucks, but these are probably the most beneficial topics you can discuss with your a pre-travel provider.

and Turkey are 23 and 44, respectively—meaning that per mile traveled, you are 21 times more likely to die on the road in Sri Lanka, and 40 times more likely in Turkey. So does Turkey have the worst roads in the world? Not even close. Turkey, to its credit, collects accurate statistics. In many countries there is no official tally. In Ghana, for example, only about 10% of road fatalities are tallied by officials. So does Ghana have the worst roads in the world? No! Ghana has stable government. Wars and other causes of societal disruption are always associated with an increase in road traffic fatalities. Collapsing or failed states, such as Somalia, undoubtedly have rates of road traffic fatalities that are astronomical. No one knows the true figures.

The pattern of fatalities differs between developed and developing counties. In the US, over 60% of road traffic accident fatalities occur in drivers; in the developing world, fewer than 10% of fatalities occur in drivers. Urban pedestrians alone account for about 65% of auto-related deaths in poor countries.

There are many, many reasons that road traffic accidents are more common in the developing world. The roads are bad, cars are in poor condition, people do not follow the laws, the laws are not enforced, people ride in creative places such as the roofs of buses and the backs of open trucks, kids don't ride in car seats, vehicles do not have seat belts, and people do not use them if they do.

And folks in the developing world seem prone to tippling, then driving. The percentage of drivers with blood alcohol levels higher than 80 mg/dl, indicating impairment, has been found to be 0.4% in Denmark, 3.4% in France—and 21% in Accra, the capital of Ghana. And alarmingly, 4% of bus drivers and 8% of truck drivers in Ghana were found to have blood alcohol levels above this level.

Compounding the high rate of accidents, there is no formal

emergency medical system in most developing countries. If you crash your car in the developing world, you do not call 911—there is no operator standing by. You hitchhike, taxi, walk, or crawl to the nearest medical facility, which, if you are in a rural area, may consist of little more than a well-intentioned village healer. Research shows that your odds of dying from a life-threatening injury are markedly higher in the developing world—36%, as opposed to 6% in the developed world in one study.

And, not surprisingly, this translates into a higher rate of death via road traffic accidents in tourists. Male travelers between fifteen and forty-four years of age have a two to three times higher rate of death in the developing world as compared with the same age group in developed nations.

REDUCING ROAD TRAFFIC RISK

+ Most important: Seat belts are good. There is no single intervention in a motor vehicle that will raise your odds of surviving a crash as dramatically as will wearing a seat belt. Lap and shoulder both are best, but using a lap belt only yields significant benefits.
+ Avoid renting anything motorized and two-wheeled. If you do, wear a helmet. If you ride a bike, wear a helmet. Do not ride as a passenger without a helmet.
+ Avoid road travel at night. For some reason, truck drivers in the developing world like to drive with their headlights off at night, even when their trucks have lights that work just fine. Someone told me this is because of a belief that using headlights at night will run the battery down. Between these unilluminated yet high-speed trucks, livestock on the road, pedestrians on the road, crashes on the road—it makes sense to limit your road time to daylight hours.

+ Avoid the back of an open truck, the roof of a bus, or other "informal" riding locations. If you are in the back of a truck, or on the roof of a bus, and that truck or bus suddenly turns or stops, you become a "missile"; that is, you become airborne until you strike something sufficiently solid to stop you, such as a tree. The tree will do well, you will do poorly. Ride inside the vehicle.
+ Don't be macho. So some guy cuts you off? Let him. So some car passes you even though you are driving the superior vehicle? So what. Derive your sense of self-worth from some other avenue than besting other motorists.
+ Remember what your parents told you when you were five? *Look both ways.* A significant number of crashes—car vs. car, and car vs. pedestrian—occur because people mix up what side of the road to drive on.

Winston Churchill fought in six wars and was taken prisoner of war in South Africa. And where did the sole traumatic injury of his life occur? New York City. In 1931, near New York City's Central Park, Churchill looked right to check for traffic as he stepped into the street, and was struck by a taxi. He sustained a scalp laceration down to the skull and two fractured ribs, and was hospitalized for a week. Even on one-way roads, even if you do not hear a car: Look both ways before stepping into the street. Similarly, if you are driving in a country in which cars drive on the side of the road opposite to the side you're accustomed to, it would not be overkill to place a handwritten note to yourself on the dashboard, e.g., Drive on the left!

Now, if you've spent significant time in the developing world, you will immediately see a problem with my advice. The truth is that many—most?—cars in the developing world do not have seat belts. However, if you find a taxi with a seat belt, ask that guy to come to your hotel the next morning when you think you'll need a taxi. I advise helmets for cyclists—many rental places do not stock them. If you are renting a car in advance, ask the rental agency if all their cars have seat belts. If you plan on renting a bicycle, take a helmet. I advise that you do not rent anything motorized and two-wheeled; if you do, do not even think of starting off without a helmet.

So what should you do about this high rate of crashes? I've just told you that roads are markedly less safe than those in developed nations and that road traffic accidents are the number one killer of nonelderly international travelers. Should you just cross all those unwealthy nations off your itinerary?

Well, it's your call—but here's my take. If you do poorly with shades-of-gray discussion, best skip ahead to the next section. My thought is that, in essence, it's worth it. Even taking this high rate of road traffic accidents into account, recall that only 1 in 100,000 international travelers dies abroad. The vast majority of people who travel in the developing world return home intact and yearning for more travel in the developing world. Yes, the roads are more dangerous, but you can tweak the odds in the right direction by following the above advice.

DROWNING

Drowning is second only to motor vehicle accidents as a cause of accidental death in international travelers: about 15% of all deaths of travelers are due to drowning. Interestingly, treatment in an intensive care unit (ICU) or medical unit has little effect on the outcome of those admitted to hospitals following drowning injuries; hence prevention is paramount.

+ Bring and use a personal flotation device if you're going to be about water—this is particularly important if you can't swim.
+ Learn to swim.
+ If you have more than one alcoholic drink, stay out of the water.
+ Your first entry into any body of water should be feet-first. Assuming that water is sufficiently deep to dive head-first into can cause paralysis or death if the water is shallow.

OTHER CAUSES OF ACCIDENTS AND TRAUMA

It is not only cars that can do you harm in a developing world city. Recently I saw a college student with a sinus infection at my clinic. As we chatted, I noted several large healed surgical scars over his left elbow. I asked what had happened, and he said that two years prior he visited Istanbul, Turkey, and stepped into an old-style cage elevator in an office building. Momentarily distracted, he allowed the cage door to close on his arm. He couldn't free his arm. The elevator then changed floors. He was lucky that his arm wasn't amputated. Take-home message: While abroad, low-level ongoing vigilance is good. Precipices will not be marked; you may see a springy diving board over water that is only four feet deep.

And don't sit under the coconut tree. Think about it. Coconuts, gravity, your head. People die every year from being hit on the head by coconuts. Had Sir Isaac Newton been sitting under a coconut tree instead of an apple tree, he would have had no further insights whatsoever. While not a common cause of death, it takes little effort to lay out your towel outside the drop zone.

AIR POLLUTION

The first attempt to control air pollution occurred in 1306, when England's King Edward I banned the burning of coal in an effort to control the malodorous clouds of coal smoke over London. The ban was not enforced, and London became one of the first cities to suffer from significant air pollution.

You do not need to memorize which developing world cities have polluted air; it is safe to state that virtually all developing world big cities have crummy air. And when I say that developing nations have crummy air, I do not mean that their air is a little more polluted than air in well-to-do big cities, I mean that their air is fantastically worse. Some examples:

	Total suspended particulates (in micrograms per cubic meter)
Stockholm	9
Mexico City	279
Lanzhou, China	732

Sulfur dioxide is formed by the burning of fossil fuels, such as oil and gas.

	Sulfur dioxide (in micrograms per cubic meter)
Los Angeles, California	9
Guiyang, China	424

That translates to Guiyang's having a level of sulfur dioxide that is forty-seven times higher than that found in Los Angeles, which is considered significantly polluted by the standards of affluent nations. And all the other usual components of air polluted by industry and motor vehicles, from carbon monoxide to lead, are also much higher in developing world big cities.

In 1992 Mexico City was designated by the World Health Organization as having the most polluted air in the world. However, through regulatory control, the air in Mexico City, while still significantly polluted, is much improved. Currently China has the unwelcome distinction of having nine of the ten most polluted cities in the world. Air pollution in Asia will probably get worse before it gets better: the number of vehicles in many Asian big cities, including Delhi and Manila, has been doubling every seven years.

If you're young and fit, breathing bad smog for a few days is unlikely to cause anything worse than stinging eyes, a cough, and a sore chest. However, some people's asthma is made worse by smog. The folks who can really get into trouble with smog are: 1) the elderly, and 2) those with pre-existing cardiac or pulmonary conditions.

Smog contains, among other noxious chemicals, carbon monoxide. Carbon monoxide binds to the hemoglobin in your red blood cells with a much greater affinity than does oxygen. The net result is that your blood is less able to carry oxygen to your body. The "carboxyhemoglobin level" is that percentage of your red blood cells' hemoglobin that is attached not to oxygen, but to carbon monoxide. People with chronic cardiac disease (e.g., coronary artery disease) or pulmonary problems (e.g., chronic bronchitis or emphysema) may develop angina or shortness of breath at a carboxyhemoglobin level of 3 to 4%. Vigorous exercise in a heavily polluted city can raise the carboxyhemoglobin level to 5% within ninety minutes. Additionally, elevated carbon monoxide levels have been shown to increase the rates of hospitalization for people with a history of congestive heart failure.

Both long-term and short-term studies have found that a number of constituents of smoggy air, including ozone and particulates, correspond to both hospital admissions and deaths.

Long-term exposure to ozone raises the risk of developing

asthma; short-term exposure to ozone causes increased risk of pneumonia and exacerbations of asthma and chronic obstructive pulmonary disease. And of course, as with smoking, long-term exposure to several components of smog will raise your risk of lung and other cancers. However, virtually all of the research that has been done on the health effects of smog have concentrated on long-term residents of polluted regions; our thoughts regarding the effect of air pollution on travelers are based on extrapolation and guesswork.

What does all this mean for the international traveler? People with a history of asthma that has been made worse by air pollution will obviously want to minimize their exposure to polluted cities. In addition, it would be prudent for people with asthma to travel with an additional inhaler, and an oral steroid, such as prednisone or methylprednisolone (Medrol dose-pack), for as-needed use. Travelers with a history of chronic obstructive pulmonary disease (either chronic bronchitis or emphysema) should carry, in addition to their usual medications, a three-drug "rescue cocktail," for exacerbations, consisting of an additional inhaler, an appropriate antibiotic, and an oral steroid. Travelers with shortness of breath that is not quickly improved with those additional medications should have a very low threshold for seeking medical care.

Prior to travel, elderly travelers may want to consider getting a physical exam with stress treadmill and pulmonary function testing. Certainly travelers with known cardiac or pulmonary disease will want to have those conditions under good control prior to their departure.

Travelers with a history of cardiac or pulmonary disease may want to minimize their duration of stay in heavily polluted cities and avoid heavy exercise while residing therein. For some, airport transfer only may be the wiser option.

Cities, like mountains, are capable of creating their own weather. Asphalt and concrete absorb light, then reradiate it as infrared radiation, raising the temperature. Termed the "urban heat island effect," this infrared radiation often raises city temperature 2 to 10° F. For example, the population of the Phoenix valley region grew over tenfold between 1944 and 1984, from 150,000 to 1.8 million; during that period its average summertime lows increased by 8° F. Every year, hundreds of people in the US are killed by heat illness; the elderly are particularly at risk. The risk for women seems to be somewhat greater than that for men.

"Thermoregulation" is our bodies' method of keeping us cool in hot places and warm in cool places. Thermoregulation is impaired by a variety of factors, including a number of drugs, e.g., phenothiazines, anticholinergics, diuretics, beta-blockers, and alcohol (see table below.)

At rest, our temperature doesn't vary much: about plus or minus 0.3 degrees C (half a degree F) at rest. This increases up to 2 degrees C (3.6 degrees F) in more extreme temperatures while exercising.

Ordinarily, sweat cools us down. It's hot, we sweat, the sweat evaporates, we feel cooler. However, when the humidity is high, sweat does not work: you sweat, it does not evaporate, you do not feel cooler. In high humidity sweating only leads to fluid loss.

Over 230 years ago, Scottish physician James Lind wrote that habituation to hot climates leads to a lessened risk to health; this has been borne out by modern research. After several days in a hot climate, core body temperature and heart rate become less elevated, the ability to sweat increases, and the concentration of salt in sweat drops to one-third of what it is in the nonacclimatized.

Drinking a lot of fluids is a good idea. Do not rely on thirst to tell you that you need to drink more water. It's really hot and you've drunk eight liters of water and you haven't had to urinate for six hours and you feel fine? That means you need to drink more water. Drink water to the point that your urine is close to colorless. Use the marathoner's rule: dark yellow urine = drink more water.

Avoiding the midday sun is smart. In hot environs you may want to live a crepuscular lifestyle: most active at dawn and dusk. There is wisdom in the Latin American custom of *la siesta*—the afternoon nap.

Drugs That Can Impair Thermoregulation and Make You More Susceptible to Heat Illness

Category	Examples
Phenothiazines	Phenergan (promethazine)
	Compazine (prochloroperazine)
	Thorazine (chlorpromazine)
Anticholinergics	Bentyl (dicyclomine)
	Lomotil (diphenoxylate and atropine)
	Levsin, Levbid (hyoscyamine)
	Transderm-Scop (scopolamine)
	Artane (trihexyphenidyl)
	Cogentin (benztropine)
	Benadryl* (diphenhydramine)
Diuretics	hydrochlorothiazide
	chlorthalidone
	trichlormethiazide
Beta-blockers	metopolol
	propranolol
Alcoholic beverages	Budweiser

* Note: Benadryl is both an anticholinergic and an antihistamine.

Having sex with a new partner while abroad is common. In one Spanish study, 19% of international travelers had a new sexual partner while abroad, and only about half used condoms. Alarmingly, a high percentage—3.4%—of those who did not use condoms acquired HIV infection. An Australian study showed that only one in three travelers would *not* have sex with a new partner should an opportunity arise. (I'm not implying that the Australians are a particularly randy people; I think the figures would be similar for any industrialized country.) Overall, studies show that between one-quarter and one-third of travelers sleep with someone new while abroad.

The likelihood of having a new partner while abroad is higher in men, in those traveling without their usual partner, and with increasing duration of stay. In a study of 1,200 Peace Corps volunteers, 60% had sex with another Peace Corps volunteer and 39% reported sex with a host country national. Of those who had a new partner while abroad, only 32% used condoms consistently. The typical "sex tourist"—someone who travels for the express purpose of hiring commercial sex workers—is male, with an average age of thirty-eight. A majority do not use condoms.

Not surprisingly, the risk of acquiring HIV is markedly higher while abroad. One UK study showed that the risk of international travelers was 300-fold higher while abroad compared with their at-home risk. The prevalence of HIV in commercial sex workers often exceeds 50%; in many studies it is well over 80%.

And of course HIV is only one of many afflictions you can pick up via your sex life. Gonorrhea, chlamydia, herpes, syphilis, venereal warts, and hepatitis B are among the many infections that are STDs (sexually transmitted diseases). (I could go on. Some of the more disturbing photos I have viewed during my study of tropical medicine are photos of men's and women's genitals with a variety of infections: granuloma inguinale, lymphogranuloma venereum, and chancroid. You do not want a photo of your privates grossing out a group of doctors in training.)

As to whether or not you have a new partner in your sex life while abroad, that's your business. But sleeping with someone new without using a condom is dangerous.

CRIME AND SECURITY

Although usually not a health issue per se, crime in many developing world cities, as in many cities in the developed world, is common. International travelers may be viewed as walking automated teller machines. The math isn't complex: they're poor, you're rich. Do not carry your valuables in a fanny pack ("bum bag" in UK parlance). These are easy targets for thieves. Carry one if you want, but only keep lunch and trinket money in it.

Beware the mustard scam, in which someone sprays something on your clothes, then helps you by wiping it off as they help themselves to whatever they can find in your pockets. If someone points out something on your clothes—keep walking. Some thieves prefer the slash 'n' grab technique, in which the bottom of your bag is slashed with a very sharp knife, and the crook grabs whatever falls out.

And of course, if someone demands your wallet, or anything else on your person, *give it to them*. Even if you are personally affronted by your assailant's behavior, even if you are big and strong and he is small. A knife or gun wielded by even a small person can send you to the sphere of heavenly reward sooner than you want to see it.

War, major internal strife, and natural disasters are not spectator events; countries with significant turmoil should be avoided.

The US State Department maintains a list of countries for which they have issued travel warnings; this is available on their web site: *http://travel.state.gov/travel/warnings*. Street demonstrations in the developing world can turn violent with little warning; you should not photograph or join in protests.

Wearing clothes with a military appearance—camouflage-pattern fatigues and such—is unwise in the developing world. Many developing nations have a history of unwelcome military intervention in their recent past, and travelers dressed in garb that strikes residents as being reminiscent of armed forces may draw unwelcome attention.

Inform friends and family of your itinerary, and carry a mobile phone if possible in regions with cell phone reception.

Do not wear shiny stuff into the jungle. Monkeys and birds can be attracted to shiny things, such as necklaces, bracelets, and earrings. You do not want monkeys or birds pulling your jewelry off.

CRIME AND SECURITY Q & A

Q I want to take my laptop computer. Is that a problem?

A Probably. I advise you to leave the laptop at home. Let's look at the pros and cons of keeping your journal on a laptop, as opposed to writing in longhand on a clipboard or in a spiral-bound notebook.

	Laptop	Clipboard
Price	Expensive	Cheap
Power needs	Needs electricity	Doesn't need electricity

	Laptop	Clipboard
Adaptor plug	Adaptor plug needed for most of developing world	No adaptor plug needed
Affected by sunlight	Useless in bright sunlight	Not hampered by bright sunlight
Potential for theft	High	Near zero
Durability	Can be damaged by humidity or rough handling	Nearly indestructible; not adversely affected by high humidity

I've left my writing with clipboard, or spiral-bound notebook, on the table/bar/beach unattended all over the world and have never once had anyone mess with it. Contrast this with a computer, about which you will need to worry every hour of every day.

Similarly, I would leave other valuables—e.g., jewelry—at home. Sure, take a camera, but realize that you may not return with it.

Q Suppose there is a guy within sight in a uniform with a rifle or machine gun, and I want to take photos of a bridge, or a building, or anything else. What do I do?

A Prior to your trip, learn how to say, "Is taking a photograph permitted?" in the language spoken at your destinations. Walk to the guy with rifle or machine gun (preferably not startling him from behind) and ask if you can shoot photos. He will say yes, in which case you shoot photos, or no, in which case you put your camera away. In much of the developing world, the definition of what represents a possible target of terrorism or insurgency is on the

The Old Magazine Scam

I was at a bus station in Guatemala when a kid selling magazines approached me. The magazines were in English; each was plastic shrink-wrapped. They were pricey—four dollars for a *Newsweek* or *Harper's*—but I was facing a six-hour bus ride with nothing to read. I bought a *Time* for four bucks, and the kid vanished. Later, on the bus, as I was reading my magazine, something struck me as odd. What's this about William Casey having said something—wasn't he dead? And what's this about the Soviet Union—didn't that dissolve? I checked the date. The magazine was eight years old. The clever kid had stuck the price sticker over the date.

As scams go, this one was innocuous. I ended up reading it cover to cover about three times. Actually, I can't even say the kid lied—he didn't *say* the magazine was the current issue. If I assumed as much, well, that was my doing.

Have I myself ever been the victim of crime in the developing world? Yes. Once. I won't say which country, as you might deduce that that country is more dangerous than others, which it isn't. It was at a crowded bus station. My wallet was in my front pants pocket. I felt my arms momentarily pinned, a flick in my pocket, and my wallet was gone. By the time I realized what had happened, all I saw was people milling about me and I had no idea who had taken it.

That's it, in over twenty years of trips to the developing world, in Central and South America, Asia, and Africa.

I was only a little irked. It wasn't brilliant of me to keep a wallet in a pants pocket. And I wasn't hurt. It was a hassle to cancel my credit card (which was not used—I assume they grabbed the cash and tossed the rest)—but otherwise it was a minor incident, albeit a lesson for me. I no longer use a wallet when I travel to the developing world—I keep my money and passport in a belt about my waist (under pants and shirttails), or in a hotel safe deposit box.

inclusive side, and if you take photos of something—military barracks, military maneuvers, a police station, etc., etc., etc.—that is deemed sensitive, you could, at a minimum, have your film confiscated and destroyed. I've spoken with travelers who have spent several hours with developing world military or police, explaining why they were interested in whichever subjects they were photographing.

Q This hotel has safe deposit boxes, but I don't know if I can trust the desk clerk and the rest of the hotel staff.

A No strategy is foolproof, but hotel safe deposit boxes have an excellent record around the world. Hotels have a vested interest in keeping you from complaining to local police. Your belongings are almost certainly more safe in a hotel safe deposit box than on your person or in your hotel room.

Q I heard that sometimes taxi drivers kidnap tourists.

A   This is rare but it does happen. One strategy to employ is to have
your hotel call for the cab. This will probably jack up the fare a
tad, but drivers in taxis phoned by your hotel are much less likely
to do you harm, relative to drivers of taxis that you hail randomly
from the sidewalk. And—you did not hear this from me—if you
do not have a local hotel, step into the first nice hotel you see and
ask the concierge to call one for you. Usually staff at large hotels
do not check to see if you're staying there or not. (Obviously this
ploy fails at smaller establishments.) At airports avoid "informal"
taxis but instead go to the official taxi queue.

ILLICIT DRUG USE

A full one-third of the 2,500 US citizens who are arrested abroad
each year are arrested on drug charges. A number of countries,
including the Bahamas, the Dominican Republic, Jamaica, Mexico, and the Philippines, have enacted stringent drug laws that
impose mandatory jail sentences for those convicted of possess-
ing even small amounts of marijuana or cocaine for personal use.
The death penalty remains an option in several countries, including Malaysia, Pakistan, and Turkey, for those caught smuggling
illicit drugs.

If you are thinking that you might defray vacation expenses or
augment your income by bringing back heroin or cocaine from
abroad, see the 1978 movie *Midnight Express*. Enough said.

5 Diseases for Which There Are No Vaccines

THE BOTTOM LINE

Humans are at risk for, by one count, 1,415 infectious diseases; vaccines exist for only a handful. The strategies outlined below can reduce your chances of acquiring many of the diseases for which there are no vaccines.

DENGUE FEVER

Dengue fever (pronounced DEN-gee fever; the "g" is hard) is caused by a virus that is transmitted by mosquitoes; it is present throughout the tropics. Its name derives from the Swahili *ki denga pepo*, variously translated as "it is a sudden overtaking by a spirit" and "cramp-like seizure caused by an evil spirit." There is no vaccine, and no cure. Treatment is "supportive" (rest, hydration, painkillers)—doctors try to make you comfortable until the infection resolves.

It's a crummy illness; the fact that it's known as "break-bone fever" should give you some idea. You ache—you ache like you've never ached before. Often the headache is centered directly behind your eyes, as though someone were boring a subway tunnel through your head. People say it feels as though knitting needles have been driven into every joint in their bodies. This goes on for some days. You have high fevers; you may get a rash.

So, since there is no vaccine, is this a random disease—some folks get it and most do not and you have no control? NO! You have TONS of control over this. You can bring your risk down to almost zero. How? Think: vector. Mosquitoes. If mosquitoes do not bite you, you will not get this. And how do you avoid getting bitten by mosquitoes, given that they are present practically everywhere in the developing world? Simple. The same bug-avoidance measures discussed in chapter 3, on malaria:

+ Apply DEET to exposed skin (20 to 35%, not 100%).
+ Apply permethrin to all clothes.
+ Sleep under a bed net, preferably one treated with permethrin.
+ Wear long sleeves and pants.

Any one of the above measures offers some protection; the combo of all four makes you a near no-bug zone.

Note: Travelers who suspect that they have dengue fever should avoid taking aspirin or other nonsteroidal anti-inflammatory medications (e.g., Advil, Motrin [ibuprofen], Aleve [naproxen]), as these may worsen dengue's tendency to interfere with blood's ability to clot. It's fine to take Tylenol (acetaminophen) for dengue.

DENGUE FEVER Q & A

Q What with increasing urbanization, is dengue fever on the decline?

A To the contrary, it is an "emerging disease," that is, more people—both residents and travelers—are getting it each year. Epidemics are larger and more frequent. In the first four months of 2002, Brazil's Rio de Janeiro municipality reported over 95,000 cases of dengue fever, with 571 cases of dengue hemorrhagic fever, and 31 deaths.

Q Is death from dengue fever likely?

A Usually, no. Usually you're miserable, you have the worst headache of your life, but you do not die. However, there is also a severe form of dengue, called dengue hemorrhagic fever. The mechanism that causes dengue hemorrhagic fever is controversial (see box). In dengue hemorrhagic fever, in addition to the usual misery of dengue, your blood doesn't clot normally and you may spontaneously bleed from your nose, rectum, and elsewhere. About 5% of people who develop dengue hemorrhagic fever die from it. Treatment is again "supportive"—we try to keep you comfortable while your body battles the infection.

Q I think I had dengue fever. Should I be tested to see which of the four types I had, so that I can avoid getting a second, different type, and thus avoid risk of dengue hemorrhagic syndrome?

A Good question. The bottom line is that most tropical medicine specialists do not recommend routine serologic testing in people who have had, or people who may have had, dengue fever. The epidemiology of dengue is complex. Outbreaks are often of more than one serotype, and different geographic locations have epidemics of different serotypes from year to year.

What Is the Cause of Dengue Hemorrhagic Fever?

The cause of dengue hemorrhagic fever remains controversial and speculative. There are four similar but distinct
serotypes of dengue fever. If you develop dengue fever,
you will subsequently be immune for life to the specific
serotype that caused your infection. However, if you then
develop an infection with one of the other three serotypes,
not only are you not immune, but you are at increased risk
for dengue hemorrhagic fever. This mechanism is known
as "antibody-dependent enhancement." However, this is
only one of the many causal factors that have been identified. Some strains of dengue can cause dengue hemorrhagic syndrome in primary infections. Some genetic
factors seem to predispose: for example, in Cuba, whites
are more likely to develop dengue hemorrhagic fever,
blacks less likely. In Southeast Asia, children are at higher
risk to develop dengue hemorrhagic fever, while in the
Americas all ages are at risk.

The CDC has a set of slides online that explains all
this, at: http://www.cdc.gov/ncidod/dvbid/dengue/slideset/set1/
index.htm.

The reason that this question has a complex or equivocal answer
is that in theory, indeed you could find out which of the four serotypes you were infected with, then avoid travel to areas with epidemics of the other three types. However, given the shifting
nature of dengue epidemics, this is close to impossible. Probably
the best strategy is to be near-fanatical about anti-mosquito per-

sonal protection measures (PPMs) (see chapter 3), and, should you contract dengue regardless, continue to be maniacal regarding PPMs. However, if you request that your physician obtain serology to find out 1) if you indeed had dengue fever, and 2) if so, what serotype, you are within the realm of the reasonable.

LEPTOSPIROSIS

Leptospirosis is the most common zoonosis (disease spread from animals to people). Caused by a bacteria that is passed in the urine of animals, most commonly rodents, leptospirosis is acquired by swimming in, or otherwise coming into contact with, contaminated fresh water. It is present throughout the tropics and subtropics. In people who live in endemic areas, it is an occupational illness, seen in rice and sugarcane workers, sewage workers, and miners; in tourists it is seen in those who go into bodies of fresh water. It is present in the Hawaiian Islands, particularly the two with the highest rainfall, Kauai and Hawaii Island. This illness is probably underdiagnosed, since many doctors do not consider it when they see a patient with fever and jaundice.

After an incubation period that is usually between one to two weeks, but may be as brief as two days or as long as one month, the illness starts with the sudden onset of high fever, chills, and headache; many people progress to jaundice. Over 90% of cases are not too terrible and resolve without treatment. But in a minority of people symptoms are severe, often with jaundice; these cases can be life-threatening. The illness may be biphasic, that is, with two periods of symptoms separated by a period during which the person feels fine. These people have a fever and feel achy for three to seven days, then feel fine for up to a month, then develop severe symptoms, including jaundice.

In 2000, 304 athletes from 26 countries, including competitors from 29 US states, converged on northern Borneo, an island in Malaysia, to compete in "Eco-Challenge-Sabah-2000," a ten-day multisport endurance event. The contestants trekked through jungle, mountain biked, spelunked, and swam and kayaked in both fresh and salt water. After the event they returned to their respective 26 countries and a few days later, one by one, started to develop high fevers, nausea, and headaches; several developed jaundice.

The GeoSentinel Network, an international surveillance network of travel clinics, quickly recognized an uptick in leptospirosis cases and notified the CDC in the US. The CDC found that 42% of the athletes they contacted had leptospirosis, 36% of whom required hospitalization. Those taking doxycycline for malaria prevention were protected from leptospirosis.

Other outbreaks of leptospirosis have occurred in athletes. In 1998, over 110 triathletes who swam in lakes in Illinois and Wisconsin in two separate events developed leptospirosis. As is often the case, these outbreaks followed heavy rains. (Imagine all that animal urine being carried to the lake by rainwater.)

If you are going to be engaged in a freshwater sport in the tropics, such as swimming or river rafting, you may want to consider taking an antibiotic such as doxycycline prophylactically (preventatively). The dose of doxycycline for leptospirosis prevention is different than that for malaria prevention. For leptospirosis prevention, you take 200 mg once/week; for malaria prevention you take 100 mg once/day. The malaria regimen is sufficient to prevent leptospirosis, but the leptospirosis regimen is not sufficient to prevent malaria, so if you are attempting to prevent both, utilize the malaria regimen of 100 mg once/day.

Once the diagnosis is made, treatment with common and inexpensive antibiotics (e.g., penicillin, amoxicillin, doxycycline), if begun sufficiently early, reduces the duration and severity of illness.

LEPTOSPIROSIS Q & A

Q I'm going into the ocean, but not into fresh water. Do I have to worry about leptospirosis?

A No. The bacteria that causes it cannot live in salt water.

Q I'm going to an area that has chloroquine-sensitive malaria, so I'm taking chloroquine or Plaquenil for malaria prevention. I'll also be rafting in rivers. What should I do?

A Switch your antimalarial to doxycycline. This will prevent malaria, and prevent leptospirosis as well.

HEPATITIS C

Hepatitis C is spread by blood: you can contract it from a re-used needle or a blood transfusion. Unlike hepatitis B, it is only very rarely spread by sex. It's a nasty illness, usually lifelong, and often progresses to liver failure. Currently in the US, hepatitis C is the most common reason that people need liver transplants.

Avoidance: Avoid needle pokes, tattoos, piercings, and blood transfusions in the developing world. (See discussion on needles in chapter II, The Medical Kit.)

HIV

The drugs are better but there is still no cure. Multiple studies have shown that the risk of acquiring HIV on holiday is markedly higher than the odds of contracting it at home; this is probably related to "holiday behavior," by which I mean people who vacation not infrequently have new sexual partners.

Condoms: If you think there is even a *teeny* chance of you having a new partner while abroad, take some condoms with you. These should be latex and manufactured in the developed world. There are no restrictions on carrying condoms through customs.

STDS OTHER THAN HIV

With the exceptions of hepatitis B and human papilloma virus (HPV), there are no vaccines for sexually transmitted diseases (STDs). See section on STDs in chapter 4 on Urban Medicine.

Avoidance: same as for HIV above.

LYME DISEASE

The vaccine for Lyme disease was taken off the market in 2002. This illness, spread by ticks, is more common in temperate regions (e.g., the US, Scotland, and southern Sweden). Symptoms include rash, arthritis, and heart and nervous system disease.

Avoidance of Lyme disease: Avoid tick bites. While hiking, tuck your pants' cuffs into your boots, wear a DEET repellent, and after hiking perform a whole-body tick check with the help of a full-length mirror or a close friend.

SARS

SARS (Severe Acute Respiratory Syndrome) was first recognized in China in November 2002. Common symptoms were fever and cough. Between November 2002 and July 2003, 8,098 people developed SARS; the fatality rate was 10%. The pandemic ended in July 2003. Two researchers at a laboratory in China who worked with live SARS virus became infected with SARS in 2004. There is currently no known SARS transmission anywhere in the world.

SARS Q & A

Q Where did the SARS virus originate?

A It probably jumped from a nonhuman species. Similar viruses have been found in bats and civets (cat-like animals); however, the exact route of spread to humans remains unknown.

Q How was SARS spread?

A Close person-to-person contact by coughing or sneezing. Most people were infected by family members; additionally, a number of health care workers contracted SARS after caring for patients with the illness.

Q In what countries did the SARS epidemic occur?

A It began in China and spread to a total of twenty-nine countries worldwide.

Q Did SARS spread to North America?

A Yes. There were 438 cases and 44 deaths in Canada, most of which were in the Toronto area. In the US only eight people were confirmed by laboratory testing to have SARS; all eight had visited countries with ongoing SARS transmission. None of these eight people died.

Q Do I need to take any precautions when I visit countries where SARS was active?

A No.

For more information, see the CDC SARS home page at: *http://www.cdc.gov/ncidod/sars/*

6 Travelers' Diarrhea

THE BOTTOM LINE

+ Travelers' diarrhea is by far the most common ailment of international travelers.

+ Prudent food and beverage selection may slightly lower your risk.

+ A day or two of antibiotics, begun at the onset of symptoms, can markedly shorten its duration.

As many as half of travelers spending two weeks or longer in a developing country will get diarrhea. Acquired by eating contaminated food and drink, travelers' diarrhea is usually "self-limited"—resolving without treatment—but can significantly crimp your style for a few days. I'll describe a few strategies that may reduce risk and recommend carry-along medications that markedly lessen duration once it develops.

The great majority of travelers' diarrhea is caused by bacteria, the most common of which is ETEC: enterotoxigenic E. coli. (This is not the same type of E. *coli* that contaminates meat and other food products, causing life-threatening illness.) *Shigella* and *Salmonella* are other bacterial causes of travelers' diarrhea; both of these cause a more severe form, often with fever and bloody stools. Fortunately, both *Shigella* and *Salmonella* are much more rare in international travelers than ETEC.

DEFINITION OF TRAVELERS' DIARRHEA

Physicians use one of three definitions:

+ Three or more loose or watery bowel movements accompanied by at least one other symptom, such as abdominal cramping, within a 24-hour period.
+ Production of stool that fits the shape of its container.
+ You'll know when you have it.

Ordinarily I'm a stickler for exact medical definitions, but I think that the third description above is a reasonable working definition.

Studies show that someone eating at a different restaurant every night in the developing world will get diarrhea at a more frequent rate than will someone who is staying at a home and primarily eating home-cooked food. Combining this with the partial resistance to travelers' diarrhea that is seen in long-term visitors to developing countries, those spending extended durations with families in the developing world will develop travelers' diarrhea at a lower rate, in episodes per time, than will a short-stay visitor.

STRATEGIES TO REDUCE YOUR RISK
OF DEVELOPING TRAVELERS' DIARRHEA

FOOD CHOICE

For other topics in this book I feel I'm on solid research-based ground. People who take appropriate antimalarials only very rarely develop malaria; people who are vaccinated for hepatitis A or yellow fever almost never get those diseases. However, evidence supporting the benefit of following safe food practices is scanty. The standard line is, "Peel it, cook it, boil it, or forget it." Indeed this very well may reduce your risk. However, people like me want to see studies—ideally a large number of studies—that show "safe eaters" experience a markedly lower rate of diarrhea than do "adventurous eaters." These studies have been done, and most of them show no difference between those who follow standard precautions and those who do not. Occasionally a study will come out that shows a slight difference; then again, at least one study showed that those staying in five-star hotels had a higher risk than those residing at less expensive accommodations. The take-home message is that the benefit of safe eating, if there is a benefit, is modest.

Despite the fact that studies do not show much benefit to eating cautiously, I still think it's prudent to follow a few basic rules.

The Bad List—Culinary No-Nos

+ Food from street vendors. Stands on the street—which have no refrigeration and may be using contaminated water for all cooking—are to be avoided. Food sits out for hours or days;

risk of food poisoning is high. An exception would be something that's piping hot. For example, an ear of corn just off a fire should be okay. But in general take a pass on food from street vendors.

+ Salads. It is nearly impossible to sterilize lettuce. Often, in the developing world, "wastewater"—raw sewage—is used as fertilizer. Vegetables thrive on it, but it often carries *Salmonella*, *Shigella*, and a host of other pathogens. I advise limiting your salad eating to the developed world. If your trip is prolonged, you might consider taking a once-a-day multivitamin.
+ Raw food, such as sushi
+ Buffets, even at nice hotels or restaurants, in which food sits out for several hours
+ Tap water, even to brush your teeth (despite the fact that most cases of travelers' diarrhea are transmitted by food, not water)
+ Unpasteurized milk or other dairy products
+ Ice. Freezing doesn't kill most of the germs that can give you the runs.

The (Relatively) Safe List

+ Dry foods, such as bread
+ Packaged foods
+ Well-cooked food; boiled water
+ Bottled water (sealed)
+ Carbonated drinks (e.g., beer, pop)
+ Fruits with skin, rind, or peel that you throw away, e.g., banana, orange

"Prophylactic" means "to prevent." By this strategy, you take something for the entire time you're abroad to prevent diarrhea. There are two ways to approach this. Either you take an antibiotic, or Pepto-Bismol tablets, every day you're abroad. I recommend neither.

Antibiotics have side effects. It's true that if you take an appropriate antibiotic for your entire stay in the developing world, your risk of diarrhea lessens, but you may then suffer a side effect: rash, stomach upset, even diarrhea, the very thing you're trying to prevent. Antibiotics can cause vaginal yeast infections in women and can interact with most drugs. Given all the pros and all the cons, taking an antibiotic preventatively for an illness that is usually mild and self-limiting is a poor option.

I have different reasons for advising you to stay away from Pepto-Bismol. First off, does it work? The answer is yes. If you are sufficiently organized to chew two tablets, four times a day, for your whole trip, your risk, as shown in multiple studies, will come down by about half or two-thirds—hardly a trivial amount. However, few of us have the wherewithal to remember to take a drug four times a day for any prolonged period of time, particularly as many of us are visiting the developing world to get away from a time- and deadline-obsessed world, among other motivations. Plus, there are side effects: your tongue turns black (I'm serious) and your stool turns black and takes on an odd, slimy, clay-like consistency. (These quickly resolve when you stop the Pepto-Bismol.) I suppose that if you do not mind chewing tablets four times a day for your trip, a black tongue, and weird poop, sure, take the Pepto-Bismol. But in my experience almost no one does this.

This is the option that I recommend. You carry a few antibiotic pills, and if you feel fine, you take nothing.

In olden days (c. 1990), travel providers prescribed a sulfa-based drug, sulfamethoxazole/trimethoprim (Bactrim, Septra), which worked very nicely to hasten the return to normal bowel movements. Now, however, due to widespread resistance, that drug is nearly useless. For most adult travelers, I advise a drug in the "fluroquinolone" category, such as ciprofloxacin (Cipro) or levofloxacin (Levaquin). The former is taken twice/day, the latter once/day. A fluroquinolone antibiotic is the best drug for travelers' diarrhea in Latin America and Africa.

+ Cipro dose and schedule: 500 mg twice/day, stop when better; up to four pills per attack.
+ Cipro potential adverse effects: rash, GI upset.
+ Cipro price: cheap and decreasing, now that it is available in generic form.

Note: Drugs in the fluroquinolone category, including ciprofloxacin and levofloxacin, are not approved for use in those under eighteen years of age. See chapter 7, Traveling with Children, for treatment of children with travelers' diarrhea.

However, travelers to Southeast Asia (Brunei, Burma [Myanmar], Cambodia, East Timor, Indonesia, Laos, Malaysia, Philippines, Singapore, Thailand, and Vietnam) should carry a different drug, azithromycin (Zithromax). ETEC bacteria is the major cause of travelers' diarrhea in most of the world, and fluoroquinolones such as ciprofloxacin, as I've said, kill ETEC very nicely. However, in Southeast Asia, a different bacteria, *Campylobacter*, causes the majority of travelers' diarrhea, and the majority of *Campylobacter* in Southeast Asia is resistant to fluoroquinolones.

Azithromycin dose: Adults: one gram once. Note: Azithromycin is a derivative of erythromycin. If erythromycin has given you an upset stomach in the past, it's okay to try azithromycin; its rate of causing GI upset is much lower than that of erythromycin. But if you were allergic to erythromycin (e.g., hives, swelling), avoid it.

The region in which travelers' diarrhea is primarily caused by floruoquinolone-resistant *Campylobacter* is expanding; probably the next region for which we'll advise azithromycin will be the Indian subcontinent (India, Pakistan, Bangladesh).

Your diarrhea will resolve more quickly if you take a second drug in addition to the antibiotic—an "anti-motility" drug, that is, something that slows down the transit time of the contents of your gut. The drug used most often for this is loperamide (Imodium A-D), taken thusly: two pills at the onset of the diarrhea, then one pill after every loose bowel movement, not to exceed six pills/day. (For very mild diarrhea, one option is to use the loperamide only, without the antibiotic.) Multiple studies show that either drug, the antibiotic or loperamide, causes diarrhea to resolve more quickly; you get maximal benefit when both are taken concurrently.

There are a few caveats, however, that you must follow if you're going to use the carry-along strategy:

+ Unlike other situations in which you use antibiotics, you stop taking the carry-along antibiotics *as soon as you're better.* For example, when I write a prescription for Cipro for a brief trip, I write for only four pills per traveler. The stricken traveler should take one pill every twelve hours, commencing at the onset of diarrhea, and as soon as things are normal or near normal, no more pills are taken. Most people improve after two or three pills.

+ Only take the carry-along antibiotic and anti-motility drugs for "normal" diarrhea. If worrisome signs are present—such as fever, blood in the stool, or significant abdominal pain—see a physician instead. If you're in some remote place, take the antibiotic on the way to seeing a doctor.
+ If you've taken antibiotics for two days and your diarrhea is not calming down, see a doctor. The vast majority of standard travelers' diarrhea due to ETEC will improve after a day or two; if you're not better, maybe something else is going on.

Backpackers and campers are at risk for diarrhea caused by a protozoan organism, *Giardia*. Common antibiotics do not work to cure this. Traditionally most doctors have prescribed metronidazole (Flagyl) for *Giardia*; however, in recent years *Giardia* has become increasingly resistant to this drug. For my patients with *Giardia*, I usually prescribe tinidazole (Tindamax), 2 g once. It has three advantages over metronidazole:

+ There's less resistance to it.
+ Its once-only dosing schedule is more convenient than that of metronidazole, which you have to take three times a day for several days.
+ It has fewer side effects (e.g., less likelihood of stomach upset) than metronidazole.

But tinidazole also has its downsides:

+ It's more expensive than metronidazole.
+ Potential side effects include itchiness, headache, and fatigue.

+ As with metronidazole, you can't drink alcoholic beverages when you take tinidazole. If you do, you'll vomit for some time. (This is known as the "Antabuse-like" side effect.)

Rifaximin (Xifaxan), an antibiotic that has been available in Europe since 1987, was recently approved for use in the US by the Food and Drug Administration. It appears to be about as efficacious as ciprofloxacin in treatment of travelers' diarrhea; it can also be used preventatively to lower the risk in short-stay travelers. It is beneficial for diarrhea caused by ETEC (enterotoxigenic *E. coli*, the primary cause of travelers' diarrhea in Latin America and Africa); it is much less beneficial for *Campylobacter* (the primary cause of travelers' diarrhea in Southeast Asia).

Rifaximin is nonabsorbed; it remains in the gastrointestinal tract and hence tends to produce fewer adverse effects than other antibiotics. The preventative dose is 200 mg once or twice per day; the dose for treatment of travelers' diarrhea is 200 mg three times per day for three days.

WATER

There are several strategies to ensure that your drinking water is safe. All have pros and cons, all have their adherents and detractors. Any of the below four is a reasonable choice. It may be optimal to use a combination of the options below, depending on your circumstances.

BOTTLED

Bottled water is available in most touristed places, even in the developing world. As long as it's sealed when you buy it, the odds are good that it's safe to drink. Be suspicious of bottled water that is brought to your table already opened—it may or may not be safe.

FILTERS

Filters clear water of bacteria and larger organisms very nicely; they tend to be less helpful for viruses, which are much smaller. However, viruses are not a major cause of travelers' diarrhea, so this is a reasonable option. (And if you use a reverse osmosis filter, it will remove viruses as well.) I do not like the weight and bulkiness of filters, so I do not use this strategy myself, but if this is your preference, go for it.

BOILING

Boiling kills all microorganisms that can give you diarrhea, no ifs, ands, or buts. Viruses, bacteria, protozoan organisms—nothing lives through boiling. And, despite what you may read, you do not need to boil your water for any duration or time—just bring it to a boil, and let it cool. However, in hotels or on the road, you often do not have the means to boil water, so you probably should not rely on this as your lone strategy.

Whereas it is true that the boiling temperature of water decreases with increased altitude, the temperature of boiling water at altitude is still sufficiently high to kill microorganisms.

IODINE OR CHLORINE ("HALOGENATION")

This is the one I utilize. Some people do not like the taste of iodine-treated water, but I don't mind it. Even if you're planning on utilizing one of the above strategies, consider taking a bottle of iodine pills as a backup method of sterilizing water. Advantages of this method are that iodine tablets are inexpensive and lightweight. Add a single tablet to a liter or quart of water and wait twenty minutes. Iodine kills bacteria and viruses. Some "encapsulated organisms" (e.g., *Cryptosporidium*) can survive iodine, but they are not common causes of travelers' diarrhea. If the taste of iodine bothers you, adding a smidge of vitamin C (50 mg/liter of water) after the required contact time removes the iodine taste.

One more caveat regarding travelers' diarrhea (one that many physicians and other health personnel are unaware of): anything that reduces the acidity of your stomach will increase your susceptibility to travelers' diarrhea. Stomach acid is a major barrier against microbes; the extreme acidity of your stomach kills almost all of them. If you routinely take an antacid, such as Maalox or Mylanta, or a medication that reduces stomach acid, such as cimetadine (Tagamet), ranitidine (Zantac), famotidine (Pepcid), or omeprazole (Prilosec), your odds of getting the trots while abroad are significantly increased.

FOOD SAFETY Q & A

Q **What if a restaurant advertises that all its foods are cleaned in sterile water? Is it safe to eat there?**

A Maybe.

Q **What about organic food. Any safer?**

A Maybe. I would avoid unpasteurized milk, which can spread brucellosis, tuberculosis, the life-threatening strain of E. *coli*, and other serious illness. Also avoid unpasteurized juice, which can transmit any number of things, including *Salmonella*.

Q Since anything that reduces stomach acidity will increase my odds of travelers' diarrhea, should I stop my antacid or other acid-reducing drug prior to my trip?

A In most cases, no. Especially if you have untoward symptoms that are controlled by your medication, I think you should continue it. There is no point in going on vacation and having every meal give you heartburn.

Q So then should I avoid the developing world?

A It's your call, but I would say no. But I would certainly travel with one of the prescription drugs that shortens the duration of travelers' diarrhea as discussed above.

Q Are there potential downsides to taking carry-along antibiotics?

A You bet. In fact, if any physician ever tells you that any drug treatment never has any side effects for anyone, get a new doctor. I discuss side effects of two drugs, ciprofloxacin and azithromycin, above, but the bottom line is that any antibiotic can cause a rash, stomach upset, or diarrhea in and of itself, as well as a host of other side effects. Most people do not get these, but a significant minority do. However, overall, most people who take an appropriate antibiotic for travelers' diarrhea feel better sooner than those who do not.

Q Is every case of diarrhea abroad due to travelers' diarrhea?

A No. travelers' diarrhea is defined as diarrhea caused by an ingested microorganism—usually a bacteria—that affects the lining of the gut. Many other processes can lead to diarrhea, including pyelonephritis (kidney infection), appendicitis, and malaria. If symptoms are present that are outside the realm of ordinary, uncomplicated travelers' diarrhea (e.g., fever, blood in stool, significant abdominal pain, diarrhea that doesn't resolve after two days of antibiotics), see a physician.

Q What if I have something really serious—such as appendicitis or malaria—and I mistakenly think it's travelers' diarrhea? Couldn't I be delaying needed treatment by taking carry-along antibiotics?

A In theory, yes. In practice, however, people seem to know when they have uncomplicated travelers' diarrhea and when something more dire is going on. Travelers should have a low threshold for seeking medical care should their symptoms seem more alarming than garden-variety "turista." But as I say, travelers seem fairly savvy on this point.

Q Perhaps I should pack several different drugs—ciprofloxacin for ETEC, azithromycin for *Campylobacter*, and something for *Giardia*?

A This would work well if you pack a microscope, culture media, and a trained lab tech, but won't if you don't. You cannot tell what the cause of your diarrhea is from symptoms. It is true, for example, that *Giardia* causes particularly foul-smelling farts and belching that smells like sulfur—but this is not specific for *Giardia*. Similarly, *Campylobacter* causes symptoms that are in general more severe than those caused by ETEC, but you cannot reliably tell which bug is tormenting you by the symptoms. I advise you to take a single drug (ciprofloxacin for most of the world, azithromycin for Southeast Asia), and if that first drug doesn't work, see a physician.

Q **Do I need to carry special salts to make up an oral rehydration therapy (ORT) replacement liquid to drink in case I get travelers' diarrhea?**

A For most people, no. Travelers' diarrhea is not a dehydrating diarrhea; people with travelers' diarrhea do not tend to get dehydrated, and simple fluid replacement—water, weak tea—will usually suffice. However, this is not true at the extremes of age. In the very young (under two years old) and the elderly, travelers' diarrhea can indeed be a dehydrating diarrhea. So very young and elderly international travelers should indeed carry ORT solution. This can also be assembled on the spot. To one liter of clean water, add one level teaspoon of salt and eight level teaspoons of sugar. Adding half a cup of orange juice or half a mashed banana to each liter adds potassium and improves taste.

Q **While I'm recovering from travelers' diarrhea, should I rest my gut? Is a liquids-only diet best?**

A In olden days (twenty years ago) physicians thought that an injured gut healed best with a bland diet: liquids, toast, not much else. More recent research shows that healing guts do very well with a variety of foods and do not need to be "rested." Rapidly resuming a full diet may actually cause faster resolution of symptoms.

Q Isn't there anything I can do that will guarantee I will not get diarrhea?

A I suppose that if you fill your suitcases not with clothes but with food and drink and only consume what you've brought, your odds are small that you'll get diarrhea. Obviously this is not a realistic option. The bottom line is that diarrhea is common and your control is finite.

TRAVELERS' DIARRHEA MYTHS

"If I'm careful in my choice of food and beverages, I will not get this."

This is partially true. You can—possibly, slightly— reduce your risk of travelers' diarrhea by choosing food that's boiled, etc., but even cautious eaters develop diarrhea. Most studies have found a minimal to negligible benefit from eating cautiously.

"If I take antibiotics for this, it will lead to me being resistant to antibiotics in the future."

Taking a day or two of antibiotics for the treatment of travelers' diarrhea has not been found to lead to resistance to antibiotics. Certainly the antibiotics are not obligatory, in that travelers' diarrhea resolves on its own in most people in four to six days. However, I find that the travelers I advise—particularly if their stay abroad is brief— find the briefer duration of treated travelers' diarrhea far preferable to the four- to six-day duration of letting it run its course. Particularly if you are trying to ride in a bus or otherwise engage in some activity that limits your access to bathrooms, briefer is better.

"It's normal to get travelers' diarrhea. When people from poor countries come to the developed world, they get diarrhea too."

It's not so. The average kid in the slums of Lima, Peru, develops diarrhea about seven times per year; this is far higher than the rate of diarrhea in children in more affluent nations. Visitors to the US get diarrhea at about the same rate as do residents of the US, that is, not often.

"If I eat enough garlic/if I put enough lemon juice on my food, I never get sick."

It's hard to argue with success, but no study has shown that these measures are protective.

"I always know exactly what food or drink made me sick."

The incubation period for travelers' diarrhea can be as little as one to two hours or as long as two to three days, meaning that when you get travelers' diarrhea, everything you've consumed for the previous three days is suspect. You can't know the culprit with certainty. It's human nature to speculate, but realize that this is guesswork.

For those with a fascination with poop and its aberrations, I refer you to Ericsson, DuPont, and Steffen's 315-page, well-formed *Travelers' Diarrhea* (Hamilton, ON: B.C. Decker Inc., 2003).

7 **Traveling with Children**

+ One of the most enriching experiences that parents can share with their children is to take them to a foreign country.
+ With a small number of exceptions, a child can go anywhere an adult can go.
+ As with adults, prudent precautions (car seats, seat belts, immunizations, and a medication to prevent malaria, if needed) will minimize the chance of anything untoward occurring.

I am a big proponent of taking kids on the road. Children who do not travel tend to think that their particular corner of the world is representative; children who travel will realize that most of us who live in the developed world are wealthy and fortunate. Children of immigrants (and recall that all of us who live in the US and Canada, with the exception of Native Americans, are relatively recent immigrants) will benefit from visiting the land of their forebears and learning about their heritage firsthand. And, selfishly, another reason to take kids abroad is that they open doors. In much of the world, you will not be fascinating by dint of having originated from a faraway land—but everyone loves a cute kid. If you travel with a child, people will talk with you, open up to you, and come to your aid much more readily than if you are traveling by yourself or only in the company of other adults.

JET TRAVEL

Parents who take children on long jet rides with no planned entertainment for their kids ought to have something bad happen to them. For the very young—two to three years old—consider wrapping some favorite and familiar toys and bringing them aboard the jet. It's two pleasures in one: first the joy of unwrapping something, then—a favorite toy! (Do not try this on adults.) Also, an ample supply of water and snacks is a must. Remember that departure times may be delayed, and connections may be missed. Take more diapers and snacks than you anticipate needing. Imagine yourself backpacking with your young one(s) for twenty-four hours. What might you need? It's a pain to haul all this stuff around, but it would be worse to run out of diapers on a prolonged delay on the tarmac.

Most airlines will not allow a child under five to travel unattended by an adult. If traveling with a small baby, make your reservations as early as possible and try to reserve seats in the first row of your section. A bassinet is often built into the dividers between sections. Most US domestic flights do not require the purchase of a ticket for children under the age of two (who then sit on a parent's lap). However, most international flights require tickets for all children. Fortunately, many international carriers do not charge full price for children's tickets, and may charge as little as 10% of the cost of an adult ticket.

Travel by air is safe for children of all ages, including newborns.

VIGILANCE

If you are traveling with a toddler, get down on your hands and knees at each new hotel room and crawl about and see what your wee one might attempt to knock over, stick a finger into, or eat.

Take plastic outlet covers; they're cheap and weigh almost nothing (although those built for standard US outlets may not fit foreign outlets).

WATER SAFETY

Drowning is most common in children under the age of five around the world, in both boys and girls. A study that looked at sixty-eight British children who drowned abroad between 1996 and 2003 found that 71% of deaths occurred in swimming pools, most of which were hotel pools.

The article by Cortés, Hargarten, and Hennes in the bibliography lists twenty-nine recommendations for reducing risk of drowning. Among its key suggestions:

+ Bring personal flotation devices (PFDs) and have your children wear them when they're in or around water. Assume that your destination will not be able to supply these.
+ Close parental vigilance markedly reduces risk.
+ If you are choosing between hotels with pools, try to stay at one with a climb-resistant fence (one that is at least four feet high).
+ Avoid swimming lessons for children before the fourth birthday. A loss of normal wariness around water may more than counterbalance benefits of being able to swim.

MOTION SICKNESS

Children are all over the map in their response to motion: some are unbothered while riding in a small boat in a stormy sea, some lose their breakfast during a two-minute drive on a straight and smooth road. To reduce motion sickness while on a jet, sitting a child next to a window, facing forward, and avoiding big pre-flight meals may be of some help. Some kids do better during night flights, when they can sleep.

Over-the-counter drugs that help some children include Benadryl (diphenhydramine), Dramamine (dimenhydrinate), and Antivert (meclizine).

DOSING SCHEDULE

+ Benadryl (diphenhydramine): Dose is proportionate to weight: a 50-lb. child would receive 25 mg every six to eight hours. Not for use in those under one year of age. Available in a liquid preparation. Maximum dose: 50 mg.
+ Dramamine (dimenhydrinate): children two to six years: ¼ to ½ of a chewable 50 mg tablet every six to eight hours, not more than 1 to 1½ tablets in twenty-four hours. Children six to twelve years: ½ to 1 chewable 50 mg tablet every six to eight hours, not more than 3 tablets in twenty-four hours.
+ Antivert (meclizine): for those over the age of twelve years: 50 mg, 30 minutes prior to travel. Repeat if needed every four to six hours, not more than 150 mg/day.

Usually these help kids with mild to moderate symptoms. For severe symptoms in children over two years of age not controlled by the above drugs, the use of promethazine (dispensed by pre-

Two Boys, Two Weeks, Guatemala

In summer 2006 my wife and I took our two boys, then seven and five years old, to Guatemala for two weeks. We spent a week in Panajachel and a week in Antigua, touring coffee and macadamia nut plantations, and visiting nearby villages.

Our boys enjoyed our relaxed rules regarding soda pop (primarily Fanta Orange). Daily they asked us to buy them machetes and daily we said no. We took them to a brujo ceremony on a hilltop outside Chichicastenango. We thought they might be alarmed when the brujo, a thirtyish man in jeans and a T-shirt, pulled the head off a live chicken, but they were nonplussed and thought it fascinating that the headless corpse kicked its legs for some time.

At the end of the two weeks both boys wanted to stay longer. However, the elements with which they bonded were not those that we had anticipated.

Nate and Henry's List of Our Favorite Things about Guatemala:
5) You can ride in the back of a truck.
4) Machetes for sale everywhere.
3) Rain so hard the streets were rivers.
2) Fanta Orange.
1) They execute chickens.

scription only) can help. The Transderm-Scop (scopolamine) patch, also available by prescription only, is approved only for those over the age of twelve years (see pp. 164–65).

VACCINATIONS

As with adults, the most important vaccines are not the "travel" or exotic ones, but "standard" ones. Recall that many diseases that are quite rare in the developed world, such as measles, are common in poorer nations. Your child should be current for vaccinations for hepatitis A and B, diphtheria, pertussis, tetanus, *Haemophilus influenzae* type b, polio, measles, mumps, rubella, varicella (chickenpox), pneumococcal disease, and influenza.

The advised pediatric vaccine schedule is available online at several web sites. One way to access it is to go to Google and enter: pediatric vaccination schedule. Sites that post the current schedule include the CDC, AAFP (American Academy of Family Practice), and AAP (American Academy of Pediatrics).

Children between six and twelve months of age traveling to areas endemic for measles (including most of sub-Saharan Africa) should receive a single dose of MMR vaccine, which does not "count"; that is, they then later need to be revaccinated via the usual schedule (one dose of MMR at age twelve to fifteen months, and a second dose at least four weeks later). Children between the ages of one and four years who have had a single dose of MMR vaccine should have a second dose, at least four weeks after the first. This is a "countable" dose and does not need to be repeated at ages four to six.

REQUIRED

As with adults, only two vaccines are required in pediatric travelers to some destinations. Travelers to many countries in tropical South America or tropical Africa are required to be vaccinated for

Rotavirus

Rotavirus is a virus that causes severe diarrhea, most commonly in babies and young children. It is the most common cause of gastroenteritis in infants and young children worldwide. In the US, rotavirus causes between 55,000 and 70,000 hospitalizations and twenty to sixty deaths per year.

In the late 1990s a vaccine for rotavirus, RotaShield, was released in the US. However, it was found to be associated with a type of bowel obstruction termed intussusception and was taken off the market in 1999.

In February 2006 the Advisory Committee on Immunization Practices (ACIP) to the CDC recommended that a newly licensed vaccine for rotavirus, RotaTeq, be added to the standard childhood vaccine schedule. The vaccine schedule consists of three doses which are administered at two, four, and six months of age. The new vaccine prevents about 74% of all cases of rotavirus and about 98% of severe cases. In other words, if your child does develop rotavirus infection after the vaccine, it will probably not be a severe case. Although the new vaccine has not been associated with intussusception, it is advised that children who have had an episode of intussusception not receive the new rotavirus vaccine.

yellow fever; this vaccine is only given to children over the age of nine months.

Children traveling to Mecca, Saudi Arabia, for the Hajj are

required to be vaccinated for meningococcal meningitis. The vaccine is also advised for those traveling to the "meningitis belt" of Africa and for those who will be staying in crowded living quarters, such as college freshmen living in dorms. Children over two years of age should receive the conjugate meningococcal vaccine (Menactra). Neither the conjugate nor the polysaccharide meningococcal vaccine is approved for use in children under two years.

RECOMMENDED

Hepatitis A

All international travelers above the age of one year should receive vaccination for hepatitis A, which is spread by contaminated food and water. Children above the age of one year should receive the usual vaccine: two immunizations separated by at least six months. The CDC recommends that travelers to the developing world under the age of one year receive a single dose of IG (gamma globulin) for the prevention of hepatitis A; however, many pre-travel providers, realizing that symptoms of hepatitis A are minimal or absent in the very young, advise forgoing this.

Influenza

Influenza vaccine is recommended for children between six and twenty-four months, and those with medical conditions (e.g., asthma) that place them at increased risk for complications. I advocate influenza vaccine for virtually all travelers over six months of age. (See discussion under influenza in chapter 2.)

Typhoid Fever

Typhoid fever, spread by contaminated food and beverages, is present throughout the developing world; risk to travelers is greatest in the Indian subcontinent. It is particularly important for children who will be spending a long duration (i.e., over one month) in the developing world or who will be in remote or particularly rustic or rural environs (e.g., small villages or camping) to receive this vaccine. Although not common in international travelers, it has been contracted by even short-stay visitors. As with adults, the vaccine comes in two forms: a shot (approved down to age two years, which provides protection for two years); and four pills (approved for use in children above the age of six years; protection is good for five years). The four pills are taken on an empty stomach: one pill every other day.

Rabies

Again, this vaccine is not recommended for a child traveling to a routine tourist destination (a beach in Mexico or the Caribbean) on a short-term vacation. However, this vaccine should be considered for children on itineraries with higher risk (rural stay, village stay, prolonged stay, children of missionaries or other expatriate workers).

Teaching is important. Many children have a natural tendency to pet dogs, cats, and other animals. While usually a safe practice in the developed world, this places children at increased risk for a panoply of diseases in the developing world, including rabies.

Recall that the fatality rate for rabies, once the first symptoms develop, is 100%. After any bite or other potential exposure to mammal spit (including playing with a dead bat), 1) wash the wound with soap and copious water, then 2) see a physician for treatment whether or not your child has had the pre-exposure vaccine series.

Japanese encephalitis

See discussion under adult vaccinations in chapter 2. Vaccination for Japanese encephalitis is not advised for children under one year of age.

PREVENTING TRAVELERS' DIARRHEA IN CHILDREN

The feeding option that carries the lowest risk of travelers' diarrhea in infants is nursing. For older children, the same precautions that adults are advised to follow may be of some benefit.

Children should not take preventative antibiotics, Pepto-Bismol, or other drugs that contain salicylates.

Treatment of travelers' diarrhea in children is different than that for adults. For openers, the entire flouroquinolone class (e.g., ciprofloxacin [Cipro] or levofloxacin [Levaquin]) should be avoided in those under the age of eighteen years. For children above the age of six, azithromycin is a good choice for all destinations. One regimen is 10 mg/kg once/day on day one of treatment, then half that, once/day, on days two and three of treatment. For example, a child who weighs 66 pounds (30 kg) would receive 300 mg of azithromycin on day one, then 150 mg on days two and three.

Additionally, anti-motility drugs such as loperamide (Imodium A-D) should be avoided in children under six years of age.

Parents should have a low threshold for seeking medical care for children with diarrhea. Fever, bloody stools, significant abdominal pain, and failure to improve one to two days after beginning antibiotics are all reasons to have the child see a physician.

Small children are at risk of dehydration from travelers' diarrhea. There are several commercial preparations of ORT (oral rehydration therapy) salts that are packaged in foil wrappers; the parents mix the powder with sterile water. Alternatively, the solution is easy to produce on your own: add one level teaspoon of salt and eight level teaspoons of sugar to a liter of clean water. Consider adding half a cup of juice to improve taste.

THINGS TO ADD TO YOUR TRAVEL KIT IF TRAVELING WITH CHILDREN

+ Car seat or booster seat. I have yet to see a car seat at a car rental agency in the developing world. If you have a child of car seat or booster seat age, take one along. This is the most important precaution you can take for your child.
+ Paint may still contain lead in many parts of the developing world. A lead test kit is cheap (about US $6) and only weighs an ounce or two. You drip a bit of the test kit solution onto whatever you're curious about; a color change indicates the presence of lead. If your hotel or apartment has lead paint—move! Consuming even a small amount of chips of paint with lead can lead to symptoms in children.
+ Over-the-counter medications. I suggest that you carry several: ibuprofen (Advil, Motrin), diphenhydramine (Benadryl), and hydrocortisone 1% cream. Also, assume your young one will tumble and scrape a knee, so take some sort of antiseptic wash (although soap and water are almost as good), and antibiotic ointment such as Polysporin or Neosporin. I myself am not big on antiseptic hand wipes, but from what I read they may confer some reduction in risk of food-borne and water-borne infections. On the other hand, no one has shown that use of hand wipes reduces infections while traveling.

Sugar in the Medical Kit?

I learned a good low-budget trick when I attended a tropical medicine course in Lima. For significant skin wounds—large abrasions and such—ordinary white sugar as purchased from the grocery store makes an excellent topical antibiotic. It is not only bacteriostatic (keeps bacteria from growing) but bacteriocidal (kills bacteria on contact) due to the osmotic pressure it exerts (imagine salt on snails). It's cheap, it's easily available. Its downside is that it tends to make a mess during dressing changes, and ants will materialize in a moment if you leave any on the floor. But in a pinch—if you do not have an antibiotic ointment—reach for the sugar bowl.

TRAVELING WITH THE CHILD WITH ALLERGIES

For unknown reasons the proportion of children with allergies is increasing in the developed world. A child with allergies can travel to the developing world, but a few precautions are in order.

+ When you book your ticket you can ask your airline to serve your child food without whatever he or she is allergic to, but in my experience (my younger boy has severe peanut and sesame allergies) more often than not this is not relayed to the flight staff, who do not have anything other than standard fare. Probably best to carry sufficient allergen-free food for the flight(s).
+ Pick your restaurants with care. Even in the developed world,

wait staff will often have no idea what the food contains. If your child's allergic reaction has been severe (swelling, difficulty breathing), it might be best to forgo restaurants entirely, and eat only what you buy yourself at the grocery store.

+ Realize that labeling foods with ingredients in the developing world is not as thorough as it is in the developed world.
+ As with other medicines, do not place your EpiPens and Benadryl in checked luggage; place them in your carry-on bag.
+ On arrival to a new town, learn where the medical center is. Learn how to say "allergy" and "hospital" in the language of the country you are in.

I would not forgo international travel for a child with allergies, but a heightened vigilance is necessary. The Food Allergy and Anaphylaxis Network (FAAN) puts out a handy book, *Traveling with Food Allergy: Foreign Sources of Information*, which lists medical care and how to summon medical aid in eighteen countries. This can be ordered from the FAAN web site: *http://www.foodallergy .org/*.

THE ADOLESCENT TRAVELER

Adolescence is a period of discovering boundaries and pushing limits. I think it's a great idea to take an adolescent abroad, but there may be a disconnect between adolescents' still-developing judgment and the suddenly expanded range of options, such that they can do significant harm to themselves should they make poor decisions.

Regardless of your policy on piercings and tattoos, you must stress to your adolescent children that they must not get a piercing or tattoo in the developing world, for reasons that I discuss under "Needles" in chapter 11, The Medical Kit.

POST-TRAVEL SCREENING

TUBERCULOSIS

If your child spends at least a month in the developing world, getting a TB skin test (a "PPD") a minimum of ten weeks after return is a good idea. Similarly, should a child who has spent at least a month in the developing world develop a cough that lasts for more than three weeks, a TB skin test is indicated.

SCHISTOSOMIASIS

Any child who has fresh water exposure in an area endemic for schistosomiasis (bilharzia), e.g., swimming in a lake in Africa, should have screening for this illness. This is a blood test performed a minimum of one month after exiting the endemic area.

GI PARASITES

For those returning after lengthy stays abroad, a stool "O & P" (ova and parasite) exam is recommended, even in those without symptoms.

KIDS ABROAD Q & A

Q Are there some itineraries for which we should leave the kids at home?

A You bet.

+ There is no reason to take a child to high altitude. Studies have not been performed on the effects of high altitude on children. It would not be ethical to march a thousand children up to 20,000 feet and see how they do. The travel medicine community is split on the issue of children's sensitivity to altitude illness. Some providers feel kids are about as sensitive to altitude illness as are adults; some think they are a little more prone. The problem is that the signs of acute mountain sickness in children—irritability, fussiness, fatigue—are identical to the early signs of more serious problems, including high-altitude pulmonary edema and high-altitude cerebral edema, which are also identical to the signs of a crabby or tired kid who is having no problem whatsoever with altitude. With pre-verbal children, it's impossible to tell if they only want a nap, or if they are feeling short of breath or confused. I would advise that you leave your children with relatives or a sitter at low altitude.

In 2001 a committee of twenty-five experts on high-altitude illness published a consensus statement which concluded, "Drug prophylaxis to aid acclimatization in childhood should usually be avoided." The authors also pointed out:

- There are no data about safe absolute altitudes for ascent in children.
- The risk of acute altitude illness is for ascents above about 2,500 meters (8,200 feet), particularly sleeping above 2,500 meters.
- Intercurrent illness might increase the risk of altitude illness.
- Effects of long-term (weeks) exposure to altitude hypoxia on overall growth and brain and cardiopulmonary development are unknown. (See the article by Pollard and colleagues in the bibliography.)

+ Security risks: Children do not need to learn everything about the developing world; they can learn about war and similar turmoil when they are adolescents or older. If for some reason you are going somewhere with a high risk of civil turmoil or crime (for example, the Democratic Republic of Congo), leave the wee ones at home.

+ Babies under nine months of age should not receive the vaccine for yellow fever, hence babies under nine months should avoid travel to regions in tropical South America and tropical Africa that are endemic for yellow fever. (Babies under nine months have a risk of encephalitis, a life-threatening condition, if they receive this vaccine.)

Q What about taking a child to an area with malaria?

A Although malaria may be more severe in children than adults, I think that as long as the child is on an appropriate antimalarial drug, and parents are conscientious in their use of personal protection measures (DEET to exposed skin, permethrin to clothes, bed net) for the child, children should not be barred from regions in which malaria is present. DEET is safe for children over two months of age, but as with adults, high concentrations of DEET (over 35%) are to be avoided. Both Malarone (approved for use in children over 22 lbs [10 kg]) and mefloquine (no lower limit on age) are approved for children. Doxycycline may be used in children eight years and older. The psychiatric side effects of mefloquine occur less commonly in children. Doses are available at http://www.cdc.gov.

Store all medications, including antimalarials, on a high shelf, in childproof containers. Consuming an overdose of antimalarial medication can cause severe illness or death in small children.

Q What's the deal with ear infections and jet travel?

A Worries about eardrums of kids with ear infections rupturing during jet travel have been shown to be unfounded. However, ear pain in children with upper respiratory infections can certainly worsen during air travel. (Recall the air inside a jet is not pressurized to the equivalent of sea level, but to about 6,000 to 8,000 feet.) Premedication with acetaminophen (Tylenol) or ibuprofen (Motrin) will help minimize discomfort and crying.

Q What about taking a car seat and using it on the jet?

A The Federal Aviation Administration (FAA) "strongly recommends" the use of a car seat (they don't call them car seats [or jet seats]; they call them "child restraint systems [CRSs]").

WEIGHT OF CHILD

+ under 20 lbs: use a rear-facing CRS
+ 20 to 40 lbs: use a forward-facing CRS
+ over 40 lbs: OK to use aircraft seat belt

All car seats manufactured after January 1, 1981, have been found to be acceptable for jet travel. Your CRS should have "This restraint is certified for use in motor vehicles and aircraft" printed on it. You may be required to check car seats without this statement printed on them as baggage.

Check out the FAA site "Tips for Safe Travel with Children" at http://www.faa.gov/passengers/childsafetyseats.cfm.

8 Traveling with Chronic Medical Problems

THE BOTTOM LINE

Many people with chronic illnesses travel to the developing world every year; the vast majority return no worse for their time abroad. Indeed certain preparations and precautions may need to be undertaken, but most people with most illnesses should not limit their travel abroad due to their state of health.

~~~~~~

Most people with most medical problems can visit most destinations, but additional planning may be necessary. Travelers with chronic medical problems should seek pre-travel care at least two months prior to departure. In addition to seeing a pre-travel provider, travelers with chronic medical conditions should run their planned itineraries and activities past their usual physicians. As a general rule, symptoms—angina, shortness of breath, seizures, etc.—should be well controlled at the traveler's nation of origin before considering international travel.

All prescription medications should remain in the packaging in which they are dispensed from the pharmacy, with the names of the traveler and physician intact. Similarly, all nonprescription medications should remain in the original packaging. Medications should be transported in carry-on, not checked, luggage. One strategy is for travelers to carry a full supply of medication in carry-on, then an additional 50 to 100% of surplus medication in checked luggage.

Travelers with medical conditions that might result in their loss of consciousness (e.g., seizures, diabetes, coronary artery disease) should wear medical alert bracelets which list medical problems, medications, and allergies. The MedicAlert Foundation is a nonprofit organization that supplies medical alert bracelets and serves as a repository for medical information. Their TravelPlus program is specifically designed for international travelers (http://www.medicalert.com).

It is particularly important for travelers with chronic medical conditions to have both medical insurance and emergency medical evacuation insurance. (See discussion of this in chapter 1.)

A listing of medical clinics abroad is available via the International Association for Medical Assistance to Travelers (see discussion, chapter 15) at http://www.iamat.org.

DIABETES MELLITUS

I used to think that insulin, like milk, would spoil rapidly if not refrigerated, but in fact it's pretty hardy stuff. If you can keep it under 82° F (28° C), it will last four weeks, so for short-term trips, refrigeration is not necessary. Then again, if you plan to leave it in your car in the desert in the summer—store it with a cold pack. The insulin preparation lispro is convenient when traveling as it is particularly fast- and short-acting; it can be taken at the beginning of a meal, as opposed to regular insulin, which must be taken thirty to forty-five minutes prior to eating.

If you cross five or fewer time zones or travel north-south, you don't need to alter your daily insulin schedule. If you travel through six or more time zones, altering your schedule is necessary. Eastward travel results in a shortened day, and less insulin is needed. Skipping the evening dose when flying eastbound will cause only somewhat elevated glucose, and may help to prevent becoming hypoglycemic. One authority suggests decreasing the total daily dose of insulin by 2 to 4% for every hour of time change during eastward flights, and increasing daily dose by same for westward flights. More frequent than usual determinations of glucose—every four to six hours—may be appropriate during travel, even if you don't check your glucose that frequently at home. *The Travel and Tropical Medicine Manual*, edited by Jong and myself (see bibliography), contains handy charts for varying dose and timing of insulin for eastward and westward travel.

Travelers who control their diabetes with oral medications only, and not insulin, do not require additional doses and should take their medication according to local time. Try to avoid skipping meals.

Also, realize that meal times in the developing world do not occur with the clockwork regularity seen in developed nations. Buses break down, drivers get lost, and waiters may return with food several hours after you place your order. Carrying a supply of something sweet is smart. Insulin-dependent diabetics should consider carrying glucagon, particularly if their glucose levels are unstable.

Those who attempt to maintain their usual level of good control of their glucose values while traveling across time zones run the risk of hypoglycemia. It's probably better to accept glucose values that are somewhat elevated while traveling.

The web site of the American Diabetes Association (*http://www .diabetes.org*) is a source of information regarding airline policy for carrying medications and supplies for diabetes, as are the individual airline carriers. Laws regarding prescription drugs vary country to country; the International Diabetes Federation (http://www.idf.org; address: IDF, 1 rue Defaeqz, B-1000, Belgium) is a valuable source of information regarding this. Learning to say, "I have diabetes" and "Sugar or orange juice please" in the language of your destination is prudent.

Other sources of information regarding diabetes and international travel are: http://www.diabetes.org/pre-diabetes/travel/when-you-travel.jsp and http://www.diabetesmonitor.com; the latter lists examples of specific insulin regimens.

CHRONIC BRONCHITIS OR EMPHYSEMA

Airplanes do not pressurize to the equivalent of sea level but to about 6,000 to 8,000 feet (1,680 to 2,440 meters). Ask your physician if he or she advises that you use oxygen if you fly. If you require oxygen at home while at rest, you should not attempt flight without oxygen. You should notify the airlines well in advance of your planned flights, as most US carriers will not allow you to bring your oxygen on board; you must use their supply.

Discuss your itinerary with your physician prior to your trip. Depending on the severity of your bronchitis or emphysema, your physician may advise you to avoid high-altitude destinations.

Bad smog may preferentially affect those with chronic bronchitis or emphysema (see chapter 4, Urban Medicine). Most developing world big cities have heavily polluted air. Again, discuss your travel plans with your physician. If your chronic bronchitis or emphysema is severe, you may want to minimize your stay in developing world big cities.

CORONARY ARTERY DISEASE (CAD)

As with people with chronic bronchitis or emphysema, people with CAD or a history of MI (myocardial infarction, or heart attack) are at increased risk at high altitudes or in heavily polluted air. It's all about oxygen: CAD causes the heart to receive a diminished supply of blood and hence a diminished supply of oxygen; an MI is caused when the supply of blood is so low that part of the heart muscle dies. Both elevated altitude and heavily polluted air further reduce the ability of blood to carry oxygen. Again, run your travel plans by your physician.

If you tend to develop angina with prolonged walking, you should inform the airline that you require wheelchair assistance when you reserve your ticket. If given sufficient notice, airlines can provide this, including gate-to-gate transport at connecting airports.

Travelers with CAD should be able to walk for 100 yards and climb 12 steps before they plan to fly. People who have had an MI should avoid travel by air for at least one month afterward. Those with unstable angina, or symptoms at rest, should avoid travel by air altogether.

Travelers should pack an abundant supply of their medications; some cardiac drugs, such as digitalis (Lanoxin), may not have exact equivalents in foreign countries.

It is prudent for travelers with CAD and those who have had myocardial infarctions to pack a copy of their most recent EKG for comparison purposes, should emergency care be required. Additionally, a summary letter from your physician, including results of stress tests (treadmills), cardiac catheterizations, and other studies, should be carried.

A German study of 200 travelers with pacemakers and 148 travelers with implantable cardioverter-defibrillators found that none was affected by airport metal detectors. A pre-travel check with your cardiologist to make certain that the device is working properly, and that battery life is sufficient, is advised.

See discussion under "Chronic Bronchitis or Emphysema" above if you require oxygen.

HIV/AIDS

The best measure of the strength of your immune system is a recent CD4 count (peripheral count of CD4+ lymphocytes). Additionally, it is helpful to determine a viral load; those with a CD4 count of less than 200 (or CD4 less than 15%) with high viral load are at significant risk of new infections.

If your CD4 count is above 200, your physician may recommend that you receive live vaccines. If your CD4 count is below 200, you should avoid live vaccines (measles, mumps, rubella, oral typhoid, yellow fever, varicella [chickenpox], and intranasal influenza), due to a theoretical possibility of developing illness from the attenuated virus or bacteria. Note: There is not universal agreement on the CD4 count above which it is safe to receive live vaccines. There is a consensus that they are to be avoided in those with CD4 counts under 200; similarly everybody agrees that they are safe in those whose CD4 counts are over 500. Some authorities recommend that people with HIV/AIDS receive vaccines three to six months after initiation of highly active antiretroviral therapy (HAART).

People who are HIV-positive should be up to date on their pneumococcal, diphtheria-tetanus, hepatitis B, and influenza vaccines. Non-live vaccines, including hepatitis A, hepatitis B, polio, and meningococcus, should be given as they would be to non-HIV-positive travelers. The injection form of typhoid vaccine, which is killed, should be given instead of the oral (live) vaccine.

Yellow fever vaccine, which is also live, should be considered by HIV-positive travelers going to an endemic region if their immunosuppression is minimal or absent, as indicated by a CD4 count over 200. Some authorities state that only travelers with a CD4 count over 400 should receive vaccination for yellow fever.

Note: Those who are HIV-positive should never receive BCG vaccine, which is for prevention of tuberculosis. BCG is not routinely advised for travelers from the US.

Food- and water-borne illness may be more severe in people with HIV/AIDS, and following safe food guidelines (see chapter 6) is prudent. Taking an antibiotic on a regular basis for the prevention of diarrhea is controversial. Some pre-travel providers advise a preventative medication to reduce the risk of travelers' diarrhea in their travelers with HIV/AIDS. An advantage of rifaximin (marketed under the brandname Xifaxan in the US) for this purpose is that it is not absorbed in significant amounts; hence risk of drug interactions is extremely low.

Malaria can be more severe in people with HIV/AIDS. Travelers to areas endemic for malaria should adhere to standard malaria prophylactic medication guidelines and be diligent in their use of personal protection measures, including DEET and permethrin. There are multiple potential drug interactions between antimalarials and medications used in people with HIV/AIDS. The article by Suh and Mileno, and the chapter by Castelli and Pizzocolo, both listed in the bibliography, discuss this in some detail. Antimalarials should be started well in advance of international travel so that the traveler can be monitored for drug interactions and adverse drug effects. If you are on antiviral medications, you should be on a stable regimen for at least eight weeks prior to international travel; this allows time to identify medication side effects. Some travelers with HIV/AIDS take a drug "holiday" during their travels but this is ill-advised; interrupting antiviral medications has been linked to increased risk of illness and death.

CHRONIC RENAL FAILURE

Hemodialysis is available around the world but should be scheduled several months in advance of your arrival. The largest database of dialysis centers is online at *http://www.globaldialysis.com*; it lists over 12,000 dialysis centers in 128 countries. The National Kidney Foundation (*http://www.kidney.org*) can facilitate scheduling. The Society for Accessible Travel and Hospitality (*http://www.sath.org*) lists information on travel and cruise boat companies that organize trips that are specifically designed for travelers on dialysis.

People on dialysis require higher-than-standard doses of vaccine for hepatitis B. The effect of dialysis on most antimalarials is unknown; however, dialysis does not affect blood concentrations of mefloquine (Lariam).

MULTIPLE SCLEROSIS

Although there have been case reports of onset or exacerbation of multiple sclerosis (MS) following vaccinations, multiple large, well-controlled studies have failed to identify a link between vaccinations and short-term exacerbations. However, there is significant evidence that relapses of MS are linked to antecedent infections, including upper respiratory infections. This suggests that travelers with MS should receive vaccination for infectious illnesses for which their travel places them at significant risk (see articles by Giovanetti and by Buljevac et al. in the bibliography).

Type of immune suppression	Cautions/suggestions
Recipient of kidney, heart, lung, or liver transplant	Avoid international travel for one year post-transplant. Get pneumococcal, meningococcal, and H. flu type b vaccines. Get hepatitis B and influenza vaccines pre-transplant.
Hematologic malignancies (leukemia)	No live virus vaccines* for three months after last therapy. Get pneumococcal and H. flu type b vaccines, ideally two weeks before suppressive therapy; also DTaP, IPV (polio), and influenza; also MMR and varicella (chickenpox) if not severely immunosuppressed.
Congenital immune disorders	No live vaccines.+
Drug-induced immunosuppression (e.g., chronic steroid use of over 20 mg prednisone or its equivalent/day).	No live vaccines. Vaccinate one month or more after last dose of steroid.
Hyposplenism (having had spleen removed, or having a nonfunctioning spleen due to sickle cell anemia or other cause)	Get pneumococcal, meningococcal, H. flu type b, and influenza vaccines.
Multiple sclerosis	No change in standard vaccine practices.

This table is adapted from "Challenging Scenarios in a Travel Clinic: Advising the Complex Traveler," by Kathryn N. Suh and Maria D. Meleno, *Infectious Disease Clinics of North America*, Vol. 18, Number 1 (March 2005).

*Live virus vaccines: measles, mumps, rubella, oral polio, yellow fever, varicella (chickenpox), and influenza (intranasal, not via injection).

+Live vaccines: measles, mumps, rubella, oral typhoid, oral polio, yellow fever, BCG (for TB), varicella (chickenpox), and influenza (intranasal, not via injection).

TRAVELERS WITH CHRONIC ILLNESS Q & A

Q I'm HIV-positive, and my CD4 count is below 200. I'm going to a country that requires visitors to have immunization for yellow fever (a live vaccine). What should I do?

A Ask your pre-travel provider to write a note on a physician's letterhead, stating that you are unable to receive that vaccine for medical reasons. (I wouldn't list the exact medical reason that precludes the vaccine—this could cause delays or other complications at customs.) And then realize that you are not protected for a disease that, while not common in tourists, can be catastrophic even in tourists with intact immune systems. If you decide to go, anti-insect personal protection measures (DEET to skin, permethrin to clothes, sleeping under a net) are all the more important.

Q I'm HIV-positive, and I'm significantly immunocompromised (my CD4 count is under 200). Does international travel put me at higher risk of illness than the next guy over?

A Yes.

Q **Does that mean I should cancel my plans to visit the developing world?**

A That's your call to make.

Q **Come on! Give me a little guidance here.**

A I'm serious. It's a complex topic and there's no one right answer. International travel to the developed world, e.g., Western Europe, puts you at increased risk for head colds and influenza; these tend to be more severe in people who are immunocompromised.

Travel in the developing world puts you at increased risk for, among other illnesses, infections that cause diarrhea, and again these tend to be more severe—even life-threatening—in those with immunosuppression. Additionally, medical care may be remote and/or substandard. So the threat to health is significant—but so is the reward. To see the game parks of Africa, or the Mayan pyramids of Chiapas and Central America, or the temples of Southeast Asia, are wondrous experiences. The risk is high, the reward is high. It's complex. It's your call.

Q **Whatever happened to "doctors' orders"?**

A We don't give orders anymore. We share information and make recommendations.

Q **What's your recommendation?**

A My recommendation is that you make the call.

9 High-Altitude Medicine

THE BOTTOM LINE

Acute mountain sickness (AMS) is common in travelers who ascend to over 8,000 feet; symptoms include headache, nausea, and a generally pissy mood. High-altitude cerebral edema (HACE) and high-altitude pulmonary edema (HAPE) are life-threatening conditions, the former causing confusion and clumsiness followed by coma, the latter causing shortness of breath at rest and cough. AMS generally resolves after a couple of days at altitude. The mainstay of treatment for HACE and HAPE is descent.

ALTITUDE ILLNESS

There are three illnesses of high altitude that you should be aware of. One is common and minor; the other two are rare and life-threatening.

ACUTE MOUNTAIN SICKNESS (AMS)

Acclimatization is the process by which your body becomes adapted to breathing the thin air of high altitude. You breathe faster, your heart beats more quickly, your body produces more red blood cells to carry oxygen from your lungs to the rest of your body. All this takes several days to kick in, which is why many new arrivals to altitude experience the symptoms of AMS. AMS is the most common altitude-related ailment of those at high altitude. It occurs in about a quarter of Colorado resort skiers and over half of those who climb Mount Rainier (14,410 feet, 4,392 meters) in Washington State. It is more common in the young, in those who ascend quickly, and in those who have had it before. Interestingly, while being physically fit improves your comfort and performance at altitude, it does not lessen your odds of developing AMS.

More than half of people who ascend quickly, or fly from sea level to high altitude, find themselves experiencing headache, nausea, insomnia, and general malaise; it is often likened to a hangover. This usually comes on between a few hours to a few days after arrival at altitude; it goes away after a few days if you remain at altitude (or after return to low altitude). It does not usually lead to anything serious, but it's unpleasant and can keep you in bed. Risk is reduced by ascending slowly (no more than 1,500 feet/day), taking a rest day at 10,000 feet and at every 3,000 feet of additional gain in altitude, and/or taking acetazolamide (see below).

The two serious high-altitude illness syndromes are HACE (high-altitude cerebral edema) and HAPE (high-altitude pulmonary edema).

HIGH-ALTITUDE CEREBRAL EDEMA (HACE)

A small number of people with AMS will progress to HACE. HACE usually develops a few days after the onset of AMS. It is rare below 10,000 feet (3,050 meters). As with AMS and HAPE, rapid ascent is a risk factor. Signs and symptoms include an unsteady gait, faulty judgment, bizarre behavior, hallucinations, severe headache, and lethargy—which can progress to coma and death. HACE and HAPE can occur simultaneously.

HIGH-ALTITUDE PULMONARY EDEMA (HAPE)

As many as 1 to 2% of people who travel to above 12,000 feet (3,650 meters) develop high-altitude pulmonary edema (HAPE). Sometimes it follows AMS, or it can occur without prior warning. HAPE occurs most commonly during the second night after ascent to altitude. Early signs of HAPE are decreased exercise tolerance, dry cough, and elevated heart rate while at rest. Signs of more advanced HAPE include marked weakness, a wet cough, and shortness of breath at rest; this can progress to coma and death in as little as eight to twelve hours.

Risk factors for HAPE include rapid ascent, marked exertion on arrival, being male, obesity, and having had HAPE in the past.

You can greatly reduce your odds of all three of the above by ascending gradually. If you ascend by only 1,500 feet/day, these illnesses are markedly less likely. But most of us are only able to get away for a few days, and tend to ascend with alacrity. For example, the great majority of people who want to see Machu Picchu, the Inca site in the Peruvian Andes, fly from Lima, at sea level, to Cuzco, at 11,000 feet. Similarly most of those who summit on Mount Rainier climb the first day from Paradise, at 5,400 feet, to Camp Muir, at 10,080 feet, then quickly summit at 14,400 feet the following morning; hence the high rate of AMS in those who climb Mount Rainier.

Recognition of Significant Altitude Illness

Travelers should suspect significant altitude illness in *themselves* if they have:

+ A headache and feel "hung over"
+ Shortness of breath and a respiratory rate of over twenty breaths/minute while at rest
+ Markedly decreased appetite
+ Vomiting
+ Clumsiness
+ Unusual fatigue while walking

Travelers should suspect significant altitude illness in their *companions* who are:

+ Skipping meals
+ Not friendly, when they were friendly before
+ Stumbling or otherwise newly klutzy
+ Having difficulty with a straightforward activity
+ Arriving last at the daily destination and being the most fatigued
+ Having hallucinations or confusion

(Based on the chapter "Altitude Illness" by Stephen A. Bezruchka, in *The Travel and Tropical Medicine Manual*, E. C. Jong and R. McMullen, eds., 3rd ed. [Philadelphia: Saunders/Elsevier, 2003])

TREATMENT OF ALTITUDE ILLNESSES

ACUTE MOUNTAIN SICKNESS

Mild AMS can be treated by conservative measures: staying at the same altitude until symptoms resolve (usually one to two days), followed by cautious ascent. Symptoms can be reduced by nonnarcotic analgesics (Tylenol, Advil), relative rest, and advancing activities as tolerated. Acetazolamide 125 or 250 mg, twice a day, also usually helps. Generally only two to three days of this are needed; after a few days at altitude your body's natural acclimatization mechanisms begin to kick in. If AMS seems severe, or doesn't resolve after two to three days: descend.

HIGH-ALTITUDE PULMONARY EDEMA (HAPE) AND/OR HIGH-ALTITUDE CEREBRAL EDEMA (HACE)

Most important, descend. Oxygen, if available, will help, as will the use of a "hyperbaric bag" (a portable bag that encloses the patient; the bag is then inflated such that the pressure is equivalent to that at a lower altitude). One type of hyperbaric bag is the Gamow bag. Dexamethasone (see section below on pharmacology) is also of benefit but should only be used in conjunction with descent.

HIGH-ALTITUDE PHARMACOLOGY

ACETAZOLAMIDE

Acetazolamide (Diamox) is a weak diuretic; that is, it makes you urinate a little more. Although its primary role is to treat glau-

Tips for Preventing Altitude Illness

+ The most important point is that you should ascend slowly. There is no "correct" rate of ascent; everyone responds differently to altitude. During ascent, travelers should monitor themselves and their companions for signs and symptoms of altitude illness.

+ Climb high but sleep low. The altitude at which you sleep should rise gradually. A conservative rate of ascent would be to take two days to get to 10,000 feet (3,050 meters), then to raise the altitude at which you sleep by no more than 1,000 feet (300 meters)/night.

+ If you have a headache, never ascend to sleep.

+ Anyone who is clumsy, confused, or short of breath at rest needs to descend to below the altitude at which the symptoms began. A good test for clumsiness is the "heel-toe" walk in which you walk a straight line, touching your heel to the toe of your other foot. (This is what the police make you do to prove your sobriety.)

+ Carry drugs for high-altitude illness (see pharmacology section in this chapter).

+ Avoid sedatives, tranquilizers, and narcotic analgesics. These drugs may blunt your body's natural inclination to breathe deeply while at high altitude. Examples include alcoholic beverages, Benadryl (diphenhydramine), Valium, Xanax, Halcion, Ambien, and codeine.

+ Drink a lot of fluids.

+ Avoid strenuous overexertion while at altitude.

+ Wear appropriate clothing; that is, keep warm.

Hypothermia worsens altitude illness. The average temperature drop as you ascend is 3.5° F/1,000 feet (0.65° C/100 meters).

+ Do not assist someone in climbing higher. If someone is having trouble climbing, it may be due to altitude illness. Carrying or pulling someone to a higher altitude may be the worst thing you could do. And don't leave someone alone in a remote or high-altitude area—they may worsen and require assistance.

(Based on the chapter "Altitude Illness" by Stephen A. Bezruchka, in *The Travel and Tropical Medicine Manual*, E.C. Jong and R. McMullen, eds., 3rd ed. [Philadelphia: Saunders/Elsevier, 2003])

coma, a condition in which the pressure inside the eye is elevated, it is also used to lessen the risk of AMS. It does not reduce the risk of the more serious conditions HAPE and HACE.

In recent years, the recommended dose of acetazolamide has decreased; the current advised dose is 125 mg, twice/day, for three days, beginning one day prior to ascent. Although it's only a weak diuretic at this dose, I suggest you take the doses early in the day (say 8 a.m. and noon); this appears not to impact the benefit, while minimizing the diuretic side effect at night, when it's least convenient.

Additionally, acetazolamide can be used to treat AMS. It is entirely reasonable to take nothing preventatively, determine whether or not you develop AMS, then take acetazolamide if you do. The dose and schedule is identical to the preventative regimen: 125 mg twice a day for three days. (Note: For both prevention and treatment of AMS, there is nothing magical about the regimen of 125 mg twice per day for three days. Some people prefer 250 mg per dose, some people treat for more than three days. If you stop the medication at altitude and symptoms reoccur, it is fine to take it for a few more days.)

If you ascend slowly (no more than 1,500 feet per day), there is usually no need to take acetazolamide.

Another use for acetazolamide is to treat the poor sleep that develops at altitude. Poor sleep is almost universal at altitude; it usually improves after three or four nights at a given altitude. Acetazolamide 125 mg at bedtime significantly improves the quality of sleep for those experiencing restless nights at high altitude.

There is one innocuous, albeit weird, side effect of acetazolamide. While you're taking it, you can't tell the difference between carbonated and uncarbonated drinks. This is unlikely to affect your life unless you're a taster at a pop factory, but still, it's odd; I don't know of another drug with this side effect. In fact, while you're taking it, try drinking a carbonated pop or a beer. It'll taste "off"—not horrendous, just not right. The side effect quickly vanishes after you finish the drug. Another side effect of acetazolamide for some is tingling in the hands and feet, and around the mouth; this quickly resolves after reducing the dose or stopping the medication.

Acetazolamide is related to sulfa drugs, so if you are allergic to sulfa antibiotics stay away from acetazolamide. Also, it can occasionally make you drowsy, or sun-sensitive. It is not approved for use during pregnancy.

Testimonial to Acetazolamide

I flew from Lima, at sea level, to Cuzco, Peru, at 11,000 feet, as part of a group of twenty-eight doctors. Twenty-seven of us took acetazolamide; one did not because she was allergic to sulfa drugs. The day after we arrived, twenty-seven of us traipsed around town, a little short of breath due to the altitude but otherwise fine. The one doctor who did not take acetazolamide spent two days in bed with nausea and headache.

Acetazolamide is available in generic form and hence is inexpensive.

STEROIDS

Caveat: Steroids should never be taken while ascending; these should only be taken as part of emergency treatment, in conjunction with descent. Recall that descent is the mainstay of treatment of severe altitude illness; all other measures are secondary. Climbers who discontinue steroids while at altitude can suffer sudden life-threatening altitude illness. Never stop taking a steroid while remaining at high altitude.

Unlike acetazolamide, steroids including dexamethasone have a plethora of side effects. You can become euphoric and make unwise decisions (such as continuing to climb at dusk). Your mood can crash when you stop taking it. It sends your blood glucose up. Long-term users see even more problems.

Steroid Recap

+ Do not take preventatively.
+ If you do suffer signs and/or symptoms of HACE or HAPE and take dexamethasone or another steroid, recall that the most important part of treatment is descent; never take a steroid and remain at high altitude, or climb higher.
+ Usual dexamethasone dose: 4 mg four times a day; this needs to be tapered down when discontinued if it is taken more than three days.

GEAR

Air invariably cools as you ascend. That, combined with the potential for worsening weather, means you should always pack cold-weather gear when you climb.

Don't hike alone. Imitate scuba divers: always travel with a buddy. Remember that guy who was hiking alone in a remote desert canyon in eastern Utah when a boulder trapped his hand: after a five-day wait he performed an amputation at the forearm to escape. Had he been hiking with a buddy, that buddy could have trotted back for help.

Look at the gear of the other climbers. If everyone else is carrying ice axes and wearing crampons and quintuple-thick parkas and you're in a tank top and tennis shoes—rethink your matériel.

Recall that who takes care of whom is dictated by circumstance. Suppose you're climbing a mountain with a doctor who gets a bad headache then begins to act weird (weirder than usual). You've just been promoted. Now *you're* the doctor. Plan: descend with the doctor, who may very well have HACE (high-altitude cerebral edema), regardless of what that doctor wants to do.

HIGH-ALTITUDE MEDICINE Q & A

Q I didn't get altitude illness the last time I climbed so I won't get it in the future, right?

A Unfortunately, past occurrence of altitude illness or lack thereof is a poor predictor of future problems. People who did fine on one climb can become ill on their next climb to identical altitude; someone who developed life-threatening HAPE or HACE may on subsequent climbs to the same altitude have no symptoms whatsoever.

Q So the biggest threats to my health as I climb are cerebral and pulmonary edema?

A No. The most common cause of death of mountaineers is falls. The best way to ensure your safety is to know what you're doing and to avoid attempting to climb a mountain that requires skills beyond your level. Rope up when you need to, take appropriate gear, including ice ax and crampons, and—as readers of Jon Krakauer's *Into Thin Air* know—adhere to your turn-back time, even if you haven't summitted. It is better to descend and climb another day than to attain a summit only to leave your carcass on the mountain.

Q If I develop AMS and do nothing, will it go away?

A Yes, usually in one to two days.

Q How can I tell AMS from HACE?

A Headache, possibly accompanied by nausea, but clear-headed and not clumsy = AMS. Confusion and/or clumsiness (e.g., unsteady gait) = HACE.

Q Can I acclimatize to any altitude?

A No, only to about 18,000 feet. There are no permanent human habitations above 18,000 feet.

Q As I climb, is there anything other than thin air I need to contend with?

A Yes, increased ultraviolet (UV) radiation. UV radiation increases by 4% for every 1,000 feet of altitude gain, increasing your risk of sunburn. Cover up and use high-SPF sun block on exposed skin.

10 Really, Really Nasty Diseases and Other Threats That Are Really, Really Rare, Thank God

THE BOTTOM LINE

All of the causes of illness and injury described in this chapter are extremely rare in tourists and other short-stay visitors to the developing world.

The next time you read about travelers being killed by volcanic ash, or devoured by a lion, recall that only 1 in 100,000 international travelers dies while abroad. Nonetheless, I will discuss a few rare conditions that you want to experience via your reading only.

CHOLERA

Outbreaks of cholera, a diarrheal disease spread by food and water, occur regularly around the world, but travelers from developed nations almost never contract this, which is fortunate, as it frequently causes death from dehydration.

Avoidance: Do not drink river water. Sad to say, but every river contains the sewage of someone upstream. Avoid food from street stands. Follow dietary guidelines discussed in chapter 6, Travelers' Diarrhea.

CHAGAS' DISEASE (AMERICAN TRYPANOSOMIASIS)

Chagas' disease is not rare in residents of Latin America; it is estimated that sixteen to eighteen million people are infected in eighteen countries in Central and South America, causing about fifty thousand deaths/year. Spread by the bite of the blood-sucking insect vectors, reduviid bugs, Chagas' disease causes chronic changes to the heart and GI tract; sudden death from ventricular fibrillation is the most common cause of death.

Avoidance: This illness is phenomenally rare in tourists. Reduviid bugs live in the recesses of roofs and walls of mud huts. Don't sleep in mud huts; if you do, sleep under a mosquito net.

KURU

Kuru is a fatal, progressive, neurological disease formerly seen in the Fore (pronounced FOUR-ay) people of the highlands of New Guinea. "Kuru" means "trembling with fear" in the Fore language. Those stricken with kuru suffered headache and joint pains followed by difficulty walking. This progressed to a tremor so severe that sitting upright was impossible. It invariably led to death within six to twenty-four months.

Epidemiological research showed the disease to be due to a small infectious particle, a prion, that infected the brain. The disease was spread by the ritual eating of departed relatives' brains. The disease was halted when the Fore followed epidemiologists' advice to stop eating cadavers' brains.

Avoidance: Do not eat anyone's brain, even if you knew them well. Remember, when you eat someone's brain, you're not only eating their brain, but the brain of everyone *they've* eaten.

THE CANDIRU FISH

The most feared fish in the Amazon is one inch long. The first time I read about the candiru fish I thought it was a travelers' myth. There is a fish in the Amazon that does *what*? Sadly it's true: indeed there is a small, near-transparent fish in the Amazon that has a predilection to swim up the urethras of animals, including people. As if that weren't disconcerting enough, they then flip their fins back, making removal difficult or impossible.

Avoidance: Do not swim in the Amazon Basin. If you do, wear snug undies or a bathing suit. If you do swim in the Amazon Basin, do not pee—they are attracted to urine.

VOLCANOES

If you're struck by a big blurp of lava, well, let's just say you won't be going through the Kübler-Ross stages of grief. In a 1999 article, researchers in Japan described the deaths of six climbers on Mount Aso, an active volcano in the Kumamoto prefecture, Japan. All six were within 250 meters (270 yards) of the crater lip when they met their end. Death was not due to lava, but to inhalation of volcanic gases.

Avoidance: Generally speaking, active volcanoes aren't subtle and are easily avoided by travelers who want to live into their senior years. Nonetheless, there are a small number of volcano nuts who enjoy getting right to the lip of active volcanoes. Enjoy volcanoes from a distance.

BEING EATEN BY A LION

A 1999 article in the *Journal of Travel Medicine* described the deaths of four tourists in South Africa who were killed by lions. Significantly, three of the four were killed as they approached the lions on foot, *as if to pet them*. Now folks, when you look at lions you may see placid animals in repose, but when they see you, they see cheeseburgers. You are food, you are prey, and you will not have time to explain your affinity for threatened species or hum *Born Free* before you become a snack.

Avoidance: At the game parks, do what the drivers do. Do they get out of the vans while in sight of lions? Or hippos or elephants or Cape buffaloes? No.

11 The Medical Kit

~~~~~~

THE BOTTOM LINE

You can't pack everything you might possibly need, but carrying a few key medical supplies reduces the odds of a late-night pharmacy run.

~~~~~~

International travelers must always be conscious of the weight of their luggage—less is better—but a small medical kit can come in handy.

Keep all medications, both prescription and nonprescription, in their original containers. Unlabeled pills in an envelope or plastic bag can draw scrutiny at customs. Carry all medications in your carry-on luggage, not in checked luggage, in case you and your checked luggage go to separate continents.

MEDICATIONS

+ Over-the-counter
  - Acetaminophen (Tylenol) and/or aspirin and/or ibuprofen

- Diphendydramine (Benadryl)
- Loperamide (Imodium A-D)
+ Topical medications
  - Antibiotic cream, e.g., Polysporin
  - Antifungal cream, e.g., Lamisil
  - Steroid cream, e.g., hydrocortisone 1%
+ Prescription
  - This depends on your destination and itinerary. For short-term travelers to popular resorts, the only prescription medication I'd recommend that you carry is an antibiotic for travelers' diarrhea.
  - Antimalarial if needed (see chapter 3, Malaria)
+ As-needed medications
  - If you need medications intermittently (for example, for migraine headaches, bladder infections, or asthma) you should assume that whatever condition you have will flare while you're abroad, and pack appropriate meds.
  - Upper respiratory infections are common in international travelers. Consider packing whichever over-the-counter medications (e.g., throat lozenges, cough syrup) you find of benefit.

MEDICAL STUFF

+ Thermometer
+ Pair of fine tweezers (for splinter removal)
+ Band-aids
+ Padded adhesive for feet for blister prevention or treatment (e.g., Moleskin or Molefoam)
+ Iodine tablets for water purification
+ Oral rehydration solution powder for infants or elderly travelers

+ Sun block. This is important. Direct sunlight at the equator is roughly equivalent to a tanning bed: if you're fair, twenty minutes will give you a rosy glow, one hour can cause blisters, six hours can land you in the hospital with second-degree burns. The SPF (sun protection factor) should be at least 15. Sun block should be applied at least half an hour prior to exposure to the sun, so that it can be absorbed by your skin. If you're swimming, a waterproof brand such as Bullfrog is best. It's best to avoid the combination bug repellent and sunscreen preparations; they tend to have too much of one ingredient and too little of the other. It's fine to apply sunblock and a DEET-based insect repellent together. When applying both, apply the sun block first, give it ten or fifteen minutes for your skin to absorb it, then apply DEET.
+ Bag Balm. I don't travel with this myself, but I've heard and read that Bag Balm (developed for cow's udders) is an excellent, inexpensive topical antibiotic.
+ DEET-based insect repellant for skin, and permethrin for clothing (see chapter 3, Malaria)

Also, something that is virtually weight-free is a copy of your glasses or contacts prescription (you can get this from your optometrist). Glasses seem to have a propensity for being sat on, stepped on, or otherwise destroyed during international travel. Most large cites will have an optician who can recreate your glasses for minimal cost. (Or consider taking an old pair of glasses as a backup.)

NEEDLES

Generally I'm one to say calm down, relax, don't sweat it, fears of illness or worse in the developing world are exaggerated—until it comes to the topics of needles and other things that break your skin. Then I'm as compulsive as can be. Put bluntly, used needles can transmit diseases that can make you sick for the rest of your life or kill you. If there is any possibility that the needle/razor/other sharp thing that might break your skin is not new, don't let it get near you.

In much of the developing world, hospitals and medical clinics re-use needles. Often the needle is cleaned between patients, but often the cleaning is ineffective at sterilizing the needle. That needle then has the potential to transmit a number of incurable illnesses, including, but not limited to, hepatitis B, hepatitis C, and HIV/AIDS.

I admit that I am probably being unfairly overly inclusive. Many clinics and hospitals in the developing world, particularly in urban centers, use a new needle for each patient. But given that the stakes are so high, I'd err on the conservative side. This should be your strategy: if a doctor or nurse or anyone else in the developing world tells you that you need a shot, blood draw, transfusion, or fluid by IV—unless you are in truly dire straights, say thanks but no thanks. Generally it's no big deal to avoid shots. Most antibiotics can be given by mouth; most diarrhea can be treated with fluids by mouth. There is in many cultures something of a "cult of the power of the injection"—and many providers will fear that you may feel that you haven't had truly good care if they do not give you a shot. If you have sufficient wits about you to be concerned about the injection, you probably aren't sick enough to need it. Admittedly, the needle may very well be sterile, and you may offend the provider by intimating their needles might be contaminated. But better that than dealing with a lifetime of illness. Similarly, I strongly advise that travelers avoid all other services and procedures that entail something sharp. You want your face, legs, or elsewhere shaved? Fine—buy a plastic blister-packed razor at a supermarket or drug store and do it yourself. You want a new piercing? Get it done in the developed world prior to or after your trip. You want a tattoo? Fine—see piercing above. Bottom line: reused needles can transmit lethal illnesses. Avoid all needles, even ones that are purportedly sterile, in the developing world.

Having said that, would I ever allow an injection in the developing world? Sure. I would if there was a significant chance that I would die if I refused the injection.

If you find yourself with appendicitis, or a fractured femur, sure, have yourself driven to a hospital in the biggest city you can make it to.

Some travel clinics prepare a package of a small number of needles and plastic syringes of different sizes, for use by travelers should the need arise. Carrying a needle package is a reasonable option for international travelers, particularly if your destination is remote, or if you're a long-term traveler.

MEDICAL INFO TO CARRY

+ Phone numbers and email of your doctors and health insurance plan back home
+ List of medications with doses
+ List of allergies
+ The wallet card that your emergency air evacuation company gives you when you sign up, with its contact information

MEDICAL KIT Q & A

Q What about a snakebite kit?

A If you are bitten by a snake you should seek medical care immediately. The old cowboy strategy of making a cut with a knife at the site of the snakebite then attempting to suck out the poison is not recommended. Dr. David Warrell, professor of tropical medicine at Oxford University, an authority on treatment of bites of venomous snakes, states that the less you do at the bite site, the better.

Those at highest risk of venomous snakebite in the developing world are those with occupational exposure, e.g., farmers. Risk is low in tourists.

Q Should I take extra medicines so that I can share them with people I meet?

A No. Your heart may be in the right place but unless you are a physician and plan on taking detailed histories and performing physical exams, you can easily do more harm than good. A few brief examples: You think a man has a head cold, and you share your penicillin. He's allergic to penicillin. He dies. You share an antimalarial, primaquine, with a woman whom you think has malaria. You neglect to first check to see if she is G6PD-deficient, which she is. The primaquine kills her. You think a boy has travelers' diarrhea, and you share your ciprofloxacin. He has appendicitis, and he dies. You get the idea. Even nonprescription medications have the potential for significant harm if misused. There is a reason that medical school and residency require, at a minimum, seven years.

12　Jet Health

~~~~~~

THE BOTTOM LINE

Below are a few tips and thoughts that can reduce the risk of a bad jet day.

~~~~~~

It is a paradoxical reality: in order to reach some remote and rural land, we must almost always first immerse ourselves in the cramped and noisy environment of the modern jet. We are grateful for these tin tubes of whoosh—without them we would spend most of our vacation traveling to and returning from our destinations—yet jets make us uncomfortable and crabby. Most of us do not hope for a good jet experience; we only hope to avoid Jet Godawfulness (delays, cancellations, hollering kid in close proximity for many hours).

JET LAG

Most of us know jet lag. You fly west or east, the sun sets at the wrong time, you feel out of sorts for a few days, then you synch to the local day-night cycle only to repeat the pattern when you fly home. Symptoms include nighttime insomnia, daytime sleepiness, irritability, inability to concentrate. It isn't debilitating, but it's a nuisance.

Our internal clock has a natural tendency to want to make our days a tad longer than twenty-four hours, and most people find that westward travel, which gives us a prolonged day, is easier than eastward travel, which shortens our day.

To reset your internal clock with bright light:

+ For west to east travel: While still in your locale of departure, get up earlier, and go to bed earlier, for two to three days prior to your trip. Expose yourself to bright light in the morning at your destination.
+ For east to west travel: While still in your locale of departure, go to bed later, and get up later, for two to three days prior to your trip. Expose yourself to bright light in the afternoon at your destination.

In fact these measures are a pain and almost no one does this.

When you travel through a large number of time zones it can take up to two weeks for your circadian clock to reset to the local light-dark cycle. Very few studies have been done on the efficacy of the various measures intended to minimize jet lag; none has been done that compares the different measures to each other.

There isn't much research on the well being of jet passengers. In July 2007 the *New England Journal of Medicine* published a study by Dr. Michael Muhm and colleagues in which 500 healthy volunteers were placed in mock jets that were pressurized to the equivalent of various altitudes. Those exposed to the equivalent of 7,000 to 8,000 feet of altitude had more discomfort—backaches, headaches, shortness of breath, lightheadedness, and decreased coordination—than did those at the equivalent of lower altitudes; these differences became apparent after three to nine hours of simulated flight. This finding prompted Boeing to recommend that cabin air pressure in its new 787 jets be set at the equivalent of 6,000 feet, instead of the more usual 8,000 feet.

JET HEALTH Q & A

Q Jets make me uptight. I hate to fly. What should I do?

A My thought is that there is minimal downside to taking a make-me-mellow pill on the days you fly. I often recommend Ambien (zolpidem) to be taken an hour prior to flights. It makes you tired, not comatose. If you take it, don't drive, and stay away from alcoholic beverages. An advantage is that it has not been shown to affect your performance—mental or physical—the next day. (This as opposed to Valium [diazepam], which can linger in you for several days.) Ambien is dispensed by prescription only. If flying makes you anxious, I think it's fully legit to ask your pre-travel provider to give you a prescription for a few tablets prior to your trip. Usual dose: 10 mg in adults (5 mg in the elderly).

Q I've heard great things about melatonin reducing or eliminating jet lag. Should I just take that to reset my clock?

A This is controversial. On one hand, I've heard a number of reports from people who feel it reduces jet lag symptoms. On the other hand, it's a hormone that has a number of influences on your body, and—here's why I come down on the "nay" side—studies are lacking. No one has taken a large group of international travelers and given them a standard dose and monitored them for efficacy and side effects. I do not recommend this hormone. I do not think it's been proven effective, and I do not think it's been proven to be safe. Given that we're talking about a condition that resolves after a few days without treatment, I'd vote for no drug at all. At some point someone may do a randomized, placebo-controlled clinical trial and show that melatonin is great stuff. But as of now, the jury's still out. Additionally, in the US melatonin tends to be sold at health food stores and is not regulated by the FDA; the result of this is that concentrations vary between different preparations, and, unlike drugs that the FDA regulates, potency may vary significantly between lots.

A recent article in *Lancet* (see citation in bibliography by Waterhouse et al.) distinguishes between travel fatigue and jet lag. The former is characterized by general fatigue that resolves after a single night's sleep, and the latter is characterized by poor sleep that lasts for several days (about two-thirds as many days as time zones crossed for eastward travel; about half as many days as time zones crossed for westward travel). The authors conclude that melatonin may reduce the symptoms of jet lag, but it isn't known if this is due to melatonin's effect as a soporific or as a hormone. They note that in regard to melatonin: "Few side-effects have been reported, but the absence of long-term trials into the toxic effects and no license are serious drawbacks to recommendation of melatonin for protracted use." They also note that children and pregnant women should avoid melatonin.

Q Where can I get more information on jet lag?

A The 2007 article by Waterhouse et al. in *Lancet* (see bibliography) provides a balanced overview of the physiology of jet lag, potential strategies to mitigate its effect, and, for the truly curious, 146 references.

Q I hate jet lag. Isn't there anything I can do to avoid it altogether?

A Sure. Instead of flying east or west, fly north or south. When you fly north or south there is no time change, hence no jet lag. Flights from Vancouver, British Columbia, to Baja California, or New York to Lima, or London to Ghana, all occur in a single time zone.

Q What about blood clots? I read that jet passengers can get blood clots and die.

A Blood clots—usually originating in the legs, then traveling to the lungs, where they can be life-threatening—seem to be slightly more common in jet passengers who fly for over six hours, particularly in those who have pre-existing risks for forming blood clots (obesity, history of previous blood clot, recent surgery, use of certain medications including birth control pills, and hormone replacement therapy). There is evidence that wearing pressure stockings (tight elastic stockings, e.g., Ted Hose, Jobst Stockings) reduces the risk of developing blood clots. Additionally, although no study has shown that these measures are of benefit, I think it's reasonable to keep well-hydrated, and walk frequently, in an attempt to reduce risk.

Q Is the air on jets super-dry and filled with germs?

A International travelers come down with the common cold and influenza more often than do folks who stay at home, so someone's coughing on them somewhere. Actually, jet cabin air is sucked through fine filters which should trap most germs. Yes, jet air is very dry, which bothers some people. Keeping well hydrated, and putting saline drops into your eyes regularly, can help to alleviate symptoms brought on by this desert-like air.

Q I have a head cold. Should I fly?

A While the odds of something bad, e.g., a ruptured eardrum, occurring when you fly with a head cold are minuscule, many people develop bothersome ear and/or sinus pain. The odds of this can be reduced by pre-flight decongestants, either by mouth (Actifed, Sudafed, Contac, others) or intranasally (Afrin). Note: Afrin should not be used for over three days due to risk of "rebound" symptoms when it's stopped.

Because security rules change regarding what is allowable to carry on, travelers should always check the Transportation Security Administration's web site, at *http://www.tsa.gov*, before traveling.

MOTION SICKNESS

Given sufficiently vigorous jostling and rocking, everyone is susceptible to motion sickness. Its symptoms are well known: cold sweats, nausea, vomiting.

MOTION SICKNESS Q & A

Q I'm prone to motion sickness. Do drugs help?

A If you have travel by boat in your plans and you're prone to motion sickness, you might consider a drug to help you to keep your lunch down. My favorite is "the patch": Transderm-Scop, which is dispensed by prescription only. You put a small patch behind an ear; it lasts for three days, at which point you put a new one on if you're still at sea. Possible side effects: dry mouth and blurry vision.

Q **What about those acupressure bracelets for motion sickness?**

A In clinical trials, bracelets do about as well at preventing motion sickness as do placebos, that is, not very well.

Q **What about over-the-counter drugs?**

A Several over-the-counter drugs have been shown to give some benefit to some people; options include Benadryl (diphenhydramine), Dramamine (dimenhydrinate), and Antivert (meclizine).

13 After Your Trip

IF YOU FEEL GOOD, IF YOU DO NOT

~~~~~~

THE BOTTOM LINE

Depending on where you've traveled, how long you've been gone, and what you've done, you may want to undergo a few screening tests after your return.

~~~~~~

POST-TRIP Q & A

Q I just returned from the developing world and I feel fine. Do I need any testing?

A It depends.

Q It depends on what?

A Primarily on the duration of your travels.

Q I was in Acapulco for a week. Do I need any screening?

A No.

Q Say I was there for a couple of months.

A Then you might consider a couple of tests. For anyone who spends at least one month in the developing world, a skin test for tuberculosis (a PPD) is advised. This test is performed at least ten weeks after exiting the developing world. A nurse places a bit of fluid under the skin of your forearm, then you return to that clinic forty-eight to seventy-two hours later to have the test read. If a bump of sufficient size appears, your test will be read as "positive" and a few months of an anti-TB medicine, isoniazid, will be recommended.

Q What else?

A Long-duration travelers to the developing world should consider getting a stool O & P (ova and parasites) test. Basically you give a lab some of your stool, which is then examined under the micro-scope for worm eggs and other things that ought not be there. Anything they can find can be eliminated with the right drug.

Q Worms! Give the lab some of my poop! Gross.

A Well, yes.

Q I hope you're finished.

A There is one more thing. There is a disease called schistosomiasis (also called bilharzia) that is transmitted in contaminated bodies of fresh water throughout the continent of Africa, and a few other places.

Q I was only in Mexico.

A It's not in Mexico. For those who have been in any body of fresh-water in Africa, we do a blood test, at least one month after potential exposure. Anyone who tests positive receives a single dose of a drug called praziquantal.

Q Are you finished?

A Yes.

Q I do not want to collect my poop to give to a lab.

A It's only recommended for long-duration travelers to the developing world. For example, part of the routine Peace Corps end-of-service exam is to collect three different stool samples for O & P exam.

Q I swam in fresh water. I feel fine. Should I be tested for leptospirosis?

A If you feel fine, there's no point.

Q What if I'm sick when I return home?

A While traveling in the developing world, travelers should keep in mind that diagnostic tests may not be performed with the accuracy we are accustomed to in the developed world. I see many travelers who have received a diagnosis of malaria while in the developing world. Well over half, when I test them, do not have and have not recently had malaria. Often these travelers took their preventative medicines for malaria as they were advised to do. In these people, malaria is very rare. If you are taking an appropriate medication to prevent malaria, and you develop fever, other causes, including dengue fever and influenza, are more likely. Often travelers are told that the local malaria is "resistant" to doxycycline or whichever medication the traveler is on. Unfortunately, this has prompted some travelers to stop their preventative medication, at which point they may develop malaria on top of whatever illness first prompted them to seek medical care.

If you feel unwell after your trip, you want to see a physician who sees returned ill travelers regularly. There is no board certification for travel or tropical medicine, but one marker of travel-health savvy is a Certificate of Knowledge in Clinical Tropical Medicine & Travelers' Health from the ASTMH (American Society of Tropical Medicine & Hygiene). The ASTMH gives a rigorous exam once a year on both pre-travel and post-travel medicine; those who pass are awarded a certificate. The ISTM (International Society of Travel Medicine) also holds an annual exam and issues certificates of knowledge; their exam covers pre-travel care only.

14 Some Tips That, Strictly Speaking, Do Not Fall under the Rubric of Travel Health That I Nonetheless Feel Impelled to Make

THE BOTTOM LINE

+ Quite often, spending less money, not more, will increase your enjoyment while abroad.

+ Travel with a guidebook.

+ Hire guides.

+ Avoid chain restaurants and chain hotels.

+ Don't complain.

+ Be a responsible traveler.

Many people travel to enter into a state that could be called the travel epiphany, or what Spaulding Gray, in his monologue *Swimming to Cambodia*, called the "perfect moment." The perfect moment is that instant during which your soul says "Ahhh!" as though it had an itchy back and someone were scratching it. Something previously jumbled aligns and you are content in a way that is difficult to articulate.

Do not wait until you are at the mountaintop, or the temple, or the waterfall, before you are open to having your touristic epiphany. Tourism is not geographically determined; it is determined by your attitude. You can see amazing things at a bus station, or in someone's backyard. You will have travel epiphanies not in proportion to your environs, but to the extent that you are open to them. (For those with an interest in the sociology of tourism, *The Tourist: A New Theory of the Leisure Class* by Dean MacCannell, a sociologist at the University of California, Davis, is a fascinating and insightful book.)

I do not know why Herman Melville, in *Moby-Dick*, wrote, "Lima, the strangest, saddest city thou can'st see." I attended a nine-week tropical medicine course in Lima and found it charming and commodious. But nonetheless big cities are not known for their propensity for extending a welcoming hand to newcomers.

The link between travel and mood has been recognized for some time. Strabo (63 BC-24 AD), in his *Geography*, wrote, "The country [Albania] produces some venomous reptiles, as scorpions and tarantulas. These tarantulas cause death in some instances by laughter, in others by grief and a longing to return home." Just as parents should pack teddy bears and blankies for their children, so should adults carry some small object able to transport them to their happy and calm places. A journal, novel, or portable cassette player can reduce blood pressure. (I would say hold off on an iPod or similar ritzy player—see earlier discussion re laptop computer.)

Realize that when something unexpected occurs, it may turn out to be the best part of your trip. There is an interval of time—call it the event-to-anecdote interval—between the occurrence of whatever odd surprise that happens to you and your realization that this turn of events, although it may delay or change your plans, is in fact a Travel Anecdote that you can share upon your return. Suppose your bus breaks down in the middle of nowhere and you have to ask a farmer if you can sleep on his floor and of course he says yes and when you wake up there are kittens between your legs and four children are watching you like you're television. Now, this may not be how you would choose to greet the day, but when you get home and relate this tale, you will be the envy of your social set. You risked serendipity, and were rewarded.

A few general rules to recall while under duress:

+ Most people are sane.
+ Most people are honest.
+ Most people are nice.

MENTAL HEALTH Q & A

Q **I'm just divorced/fired/otherwise in crisis. I want to get away from it all. Is going to the developing world a good call?**

A Probably not. While I'm a big proponent of visiting the less wealthy nations, I would not say that travel therein is low stress; on the contrary, travel in a crowded, noisy, unfamiliar country can be at times quite high stress. This is fine if you're starting off in a relatively placid state of mind, but if you're already in turmoil before you leave, I doubt that you'll find the peace of mind you're looking for. My advice: Stay home, or travel to some orderly land, such as any nation in Western Europe.

OTHER TIPS

Generally speaking, your experiences will be interesting in inverse proportion to the amount of money you spend. If you stay in a ritzy hotel in a big city, you will be very comfortable and will have absolutely nothing interesting to relate when you return. (You think people back home want to hear about how upset you got that morning when room service was so slow? Or the fuzziness of those slippers?) But if you take a bus trip—particularly if your bus breaks down—why, folks will be on the edge of their seats. You can stay at a swank place and have breakfast by yourself at a linen-covered table, or, for a twentieth of the price, you can stay at a hostel where you'll be thrown together, in courtyards and at mealtimes, with other guests. This is good if they are interesting and bad if they are not, but either way there is more likelihood of wonderfulness occurring at the hostel.

+ Buy a guidebook prior to your trip and read it.
+ Learn a few words of the language of the countries you visit. Becoming fluent is probably not realistic for most of us, but locals will appreciate even inept efforts to speak their language. Before I traveled to East Africa I memorized perhaps a hundred words of Swahili, and learned that the word for newspaper is "gazeti"; I realized that this told me not only what language that word is borrowed from, but the approximate time (Victorian England) of the borrowing.
+ Hire guides. I've never regretted hiring a guide. However, lest you think that all guides are perfect, allow me to share an anecdote told to me by my colleague Dr. C. He and his wife flew into the Mexico City airport with the intent of climbing Popocatepetl, a nearby 18,000-foot volcano. They were approached by a guide at the airport. Popocatepetl? No problem—the guide was intimate with its every route. However, a couple of days later, they were not far from the lodge at 11,000 feet when their guide (who in retrospect did seem a little portly for a mountain guide) 1) got lost, and 2) had an asthma

attack. Being a family practice doctor, Dr. C. abandoned his climb, took care of his guide, and descended with him. I do not believe that Dr. C. and his wife ever did manage to climb Popo.

But this is the only story like this that I've heard—the vast majority of guides will enhance your travels. Exhibit A: Mark Twain. In *Innocents Abroad* and his writings on Hawaii, we read that the first thing he did in a new town was to hire a guide. If you hire guides, you are following in a long and honorable practice.

If I think about the ten most recent guides I've hired—all ten have been wonderful. I saw places I wouldn't have seen without them. Mr. Liu, an elderly man who approached me on the Bund in Shanghai, took me into banks with vast marble columns and told me in some detail why these columns were magnificent. After twenty minutes he asked, "Would you like a rest?" and I replied, "What do you think?" "Good idea!" he said, and we sat on a park bench and had a most amiable chat.

Also, by hiring a guide there is a fair chance that your tourist dollar is going to the local economy.

+ Get off the bus/train/jet/boat. Although views are wonderful and it's fun to watch the scenery go by, you will invariably get a better feel for any land outside of your car/bus/train/jet. The most memorable aspects of my trip to the Copper Canyon of Mexico were the day hikes I took from Batopilas, a small village at the bottom of one of the canyons.
+ Do not complain. Try this: make a vow to yourself that not once while abroad are you going to complain. Complain *internally*—but try to keep your lip zipped if you're only going to bellyache about how miserable you are. Try to impress

your traveling companions with your stoicism. Anyone can complain, but to keep your attitude sunny when the jet is cancelled, the taxi driver gets lost, the waiter brings something totally unrelated to what you think you ordered, and it's preternaturally hot and you're sleepy—*that's* behavior that will boost your status with traveling companions.

If it's hot, if the bus isn't going anywhere, if the restaurant service is slow—keep mum. That's the way it is. You want snappy service, go to a McDonald's in your home town.

+ Avoid the chains. I admit that, buffeted by diffident or calamitous foreign land, familiar chains—McDonald's, Starbucks, etc.—can call out to you like the Sirens. Furthermore, I will not claim that I've never succumbed to their appeal. My wife and I, on our honeymoon, once ducked into a Kentucky Fried Chicken restaurant in Bangkok just to sit in its air conditioning a while.

+ Keep a journal. You might think you will never forget that on Tuesday you visited Chichicastenango, then on Thursday you took a bus to Huehuetenango. But shortly after your trip, if you are like most of us, the names will blur and fade from your memory. Plus when you write to that tall Dane who studies Joyce whom you sat next to on the bus, you can mention in your letter (feigning an excellent memory) that you recall his love of stinky cheeses.

+ On the jet that carries you from the developed world, hide your wristwatch in your carry-on. It can be surprisingly difficult, at first, to live without your wristwatch, but after a few days most people enjoy a state of lessened time awareness.

THE RESPONSIBLE TRAVELER

Travelers need to remain cognizant of the fact that they exert a huge impact on the peoples and lands that they visit. Dr. Irmgard Bauer, a researcher at James Cook University in Australia who studies the impact of tourists on the regions they visit, states that she can think of more negative than positive examples. An influx of tourists' cash often causes inflation, which decreases locals' buying power. Most of the money that tourists spend in rural areas does not stay in those regions, but is funneled toward large urban-based corporations.

Nonetheless, she has several suggestions for travelers to the developing world:

+ Use local businesses as opposed to multinational corporations.
+ Respect local customs. For example, if women are thought improper if they show their legs, don't wear shorts or a short skirt. It isn't your role to enlighten the world, at least not by what you wear. The Lonely Planet guidebooks usually carry well-informed sections detailing what is appropriate and what is not in terms of clothes, tipping, etc.

And a few thoughts on ethics and courtesy:

+ Leave a bit of money for the maid who cleans your hotel room.
+ Don't litter even if everyone else is.
+ Do not tell people you're going to mail them copies of photos unless you are.
+ If you are a student or researcher, share the results of your study with the people whom you are studying.

15 Resources for the International Traveler

~~~~~~

THE BOTTOM LINE

+ For those desirous of more in-depth information on travel health, the CDC "Yellow Book" (*Health Information for International Travel*) is an excellent resource.

+ As with every other topic known to man, there is a vast array of info regarding travel health on the Internet. I've listed a few high-yield sites below.

~~~~~~

PRINT RESOURCES

MEDICAL

An extremely useful book for travelers and medical providers alike is the CDC "Yellow Book," *Health Information for International Travel*, which is published annually. It's available free online, or you can order a hard copy with color maps for $24.95 (at *http://www.cdc.gov*; click "Travelers' Health" button to left, or go directly to the Elsevier web site).

A manual for those who want a more detailed description of tropical illness is *The Travel and Tropical Medicine Manual*, edited by Dr. Elaine Jong and myself. Although primarily aimed at medical personnel, much of this will be comprehensible to the interested layperson. Another excellent text for medical personnel is *Travel Medicine*, edited by Keystone and colleagues; see full listing in the bibliography.

For those venturing to high altitudes, Stephen Bezruchka's *Altitude Illness: Prevention and Treatment. How to Stay Healthy at Altitude from Resort Skiing to Himalayan Climbing* is readable, pragmatic, short, and inexpensive.

NONMEDICAL

The People's Guide to Mexico, by Carl Franz, Lorena Havens, and Steve Rogers, is so good that you should consider reading it even if you're not going to Mexico. Amazingly, this travel book mentions very few specific locations. It is about Mexico as a whole—and is much more informative as a result. Also, the authors' steadfast refusal to mention specific towns conveys the message that every place in Mexico, with the right attitude, is worthy of visit. The museums and ruins aren't truer, or realer, they're just more popular.

ONLINE RESOURCES

The CDC, based in Atlanta, Georgia, is the US government's primary agency that advises US citizens regarding medical preparations for international travel. Their web site (*http://www.cdc.gov*; click on button, "Travelers' Health") provides detailed descriptions of all major international diseases, with suggested preventative measures. Their data are searchable by geographic region or specific disease. The information is top-notch and updated frequently. This is an excellent place to begin your pre-travel health preparations.

Similarly, the World Health Organization (WHO) maintains an excellent web site (http://www.who.org) with up-to-date health information for international travelers.

The US State Department maintains a list of countries that they recommend that Americans avoid (http://www.state.gov). Click the "Travel & Business" tab, then "Travel Warnings." Additionally, the State Department's "Background Notes" provide overviews of countries' land, people, history, government, political conditions, economy, and foreign relations.

Other high-grade info web sites* include:

+ EMedicine: http://www.emedicine.com/emerg/environmental.htm
+ Web MD: http://www.webmd.com
+ Wilderness Medical Society: http://www.wms.org
+ International Society for Mountain Medicine: http://www.ismmed.org
+ ICAR-MEDCOM: http://www.mountainmedicine.org/mmed/icarmedcom/papers.htm
+ High Altitude Medicine Group: http://www.high-altitude-medicine.com

*Many of the web sites listed here are from the chapter on altitude illness by Thomas E. Dietz and Peter H. Hackett in J. S. Keystone et al., eds., *Travel Medicine* (Edinburgh: Mosby, 2004).

ASSOCIATIONS

The International Association for Medical Assistance to Travelers (IAMAT) is a Canada-based nonprofit organization that advises travelers about health risks and appropriate pre-travel measures. Founded in 1960, IAMAT maintains a list of English-speaking physicians around the world who have trained in North America or Europe and who have agreed to treat IAMAT members. IAMAT personnel regularly inspect clinics to make sure they maintain high standards. (I accompanied Ms. Assunta Marcolongo, president of IAMAT, on one of her inspection trips to China, and I can attest that she is thorough!) Web site: *http://www.iamat.org*; phone: 716-754-4883.

If you are in a medically related field, two key organizations are International Society of Travel Medicine (ISTM) and American Society of Tropical Medicine and Hygiene (ASTMH). ISTM, which was founded in 1978 and has 1,800 members in fifty-three countries, is more clinically based; ASTMH is more research oriented. Web sites: *http://www.istm.org, www.astmh.org*.

Other organizations include WMS (Wilderness Medical Society), which has greater emphasis on outdoor sports including backpacking and mountain climbing, and the UK-based Royal Society of Tropical Medicine and Hygiene (RSTMH).

CONFERENCES

If you are a nurse, doctor, pharmacist, dentist, nurse-practitioner, physician's assistant, or other allied health professional, there are a number of excellent conferences on travel health.

+ ISTM holds conferences, with all lectures in English, every two years.

- ISTM conference host cities:
  - May 2001: Innsbruck, Austria
  - May 2003: New York City
  - May 2005: Lisbon, Portugal
  - May 2007: Vancouver, British Columbia, Canada
  - May 2009: Budapest, Hungary
- ASTMH holds annual conferences at rotating sites within the US.
- The University of Washington hosts a two-and-a-half-day conference in Seattle on travel medicine every two years (now on even years, to be offset from the ISTM meetings). Information is available at: *http://uwcme.org*. Full disclosure: I served as chair of this course in 2006 and will be the chair again in 2008.

Glossary

antibody the molecule your body produces to fight a specific disease. The production of these can be initiated by exposure to either a particular microorganism or a vaccine. Antibodies created via either route are equally protective.

attenuated weakened. Live vaccines are made with attenuated organisms. These are sufficiently similar to the "wild type" (variety in nature that can make you ill) to cause a protective antibody response but do not make you ill.

bacteriocidal kills bacteria

bacteriostatic prevents bacteria from multiplying

developing world the poor countries. This includes most of the world, excluding the US and Canada, Western Europe, Australia and New Zealand, Japan, and Singapore. Most countries in Africa, Latin America, and Asia are in the developing world.

diuretic something that makes you urinate more

edema swelling, or fluid leak. Edema of the ankles means swelling; that is, your ankles get a little fatter. In HAPE and HACE, edema refers to fluid leaking from blood vessels into the lungs or brain, respectively.

endemic present in a particular place, e.g., malaria is endemic in the Amazon Basin.

epidemic an episode of more than usual or more than expected cases of an illness

HIV human immunodeficiency virus, the causative organism of AIDS (acquired immunodeficiency syndrome)

immune the state of being resistant to a disease

immunosuppressed a lessened ability to fight disease. Examples of people who are immunosuppressed include those who are HIV-positive with low CD4 counts, people with malignancies, and those who take steroids chronically.

incubation period the duration between exposure to a microorganism and development of symptoms

Indian subcontinent commonly used to refer to India, Pakistan, and Bangladesh; more formally equivalent to South Asia: India, Pakistan, Bangladesh, Nepal, Bhutan, Maldives, Sri Lanka, and Afghanistan

insect repellent bugs whiff it, they don't like it, they fly in the other direction, e.g., DEET. Compare to "knockdown" below.

jaundice yellowing of the skin and sclerae (whites of the eyes); a symptom of liver disease, seen in diseases including hepatitis and yellow fever. The discoloration of the skin is more difficult to detect in dark-skinned people, but the change in color of the sclerae is evident in everyone.

knockdown a chemical that kills insects on contact, e.g., permethrin, which is applied to clothes

pandemic a worldwide epidemic. Examples include the annual influenza epidemic seen in temperate latitudes and the current HIV pandemic.

pathogen a microorganism that can make you ill

prophylactic preventative

Sahel the border area between the Sahara desert and tropical Africa

STD sexually transmitted disease

subtropics the regions between the temperate regions and the tropics

temperate regions further from the equator than the subtropics, e.g., most of the US, most of Europe

tropics technically speaking, the area of the earth between 23° 27′ north and south latitudes (the Tropics of Cancer and Capricorn, respectively). More commonly used to refer to the warm regions near the equator.

tuk-tuk In Southeast Asia, taxis are most often "tuk-tuks," which are motorcycles welded to a covered seat for two. In Peru these are known as "moto-taxis."

VFR acronym for "visiting friends and relatives," people born in the developing world who move to the developed world then return to their nation of birth to visit. This group is at higher than average risk for infectious diseases when they travel to the developing world.

zoonosis disease spread from animals to people

Bibliography

"Advice for Travelers." *The Medical Letter on Drugs and Therapeutics* 40, no. 1025 (1998): 47–50.

American Academy of Pediatrics. "Follow Safety Precautions When Using DEET on Children." *http://www.aap.org/family/wnv-jun03.htm.*

Association for Safe International Road Travel (ASIRT). "Road Travel Reports." *http://www.asirt.org.*

Atkinson, W., J. Hamborsky, L. McIntyre, and C. Wolfe, eds. *Epidemiology and Prevention of Vaccine-Preventable Diseases,* 9th ed. Atlanta: Dept. of Health and Human Services, CDC, 2006.

Bacaner, J., and B. Stauffer. "Travel Medicine Considerations for North American Immigrants Visiting Friends and Relatives." *Journal of the American Medical Association* 291 (2004): 2856–64.

Baker, T. D., S. W. Hargarten, and K. S. Guptill. "The Uncounted Dead: American Civilians Dying Overseas." *Public Health Reports* 107, no. 2 (1992): 155–59.

Beny, A., A. Paz, and I. Potasman. "Psychiatric Problems in Returning Travelers: Features and Associations." *Journal of Travel Medicine* 8 (2001): 243–46.

Bezruchka, S. *Altitude Illness: Prevention and Treatment. How to Stay*

Healthy at Altitude from Resort Skiing to Himalayan Climbing. Seattle: Mountaineers Books, 1994.

Bogglid, A. K., M. Sano, and A. Humar. "Travel Patterns and Risk Behavior in Solid Organ Transplant Recipients." *Journal of Travel Medicine* 11 (2004): 37–43.

Brenner, R. A. "Committee on Injury, Violence, and Poison Prevention. Prevention of Drowning in Infants, Children, and Adolescents." *Pediatrics* 112 (2003): 440–45.

British Broadcasting Corporation. *http://news.bbc.co.uk/1/hi/health/1808826.stm.*

British Medical Journal. *http://www.ncbi.nlm.nih.gov/entrez/query.fcgi ?cmd=Retrieve&db=pubmed&dopt=Abstract&list_uids=11850369.*

Brunekreef, B., and S. T. Holgate. "Air Pollution and Health." *Lancet* 360, no. 9341 (2002): 1233–42.

Buljevac, D., H. Z. Flach, W. C. Hop, et al. "Prospective Study on the Relationship between Infections and Multiple Sclerosis Exacerbations." *Brain* 125, pt. 5 (2002): 952–60.

Burnett, R. T., R. E. Dales, J. R. Brook, et al. "Association between Ambient Carbon Monoxide Levels and Hospitalizations for Congestive Heart Failure in the Elderly in 10 Canadian Cities." *Epidemiology* 8, no. 2 (1997): 162–67.

Cabada, M. M., M. Montoya, J. I. Echevarria, et al. "Sexual Behavior in Travelers Visiting Cuzco." *Journal of Travel Medicine* 10 (2003): 214–18.

Carey, M. J., and M. E. Aitken. "Motorbike Injuries in Bermuda: A Risk for Tourists." *Annals of Emergency Medicine* 28 (1996): 424–29.

Castelli, F., and C. Pizzocolo. "The Traveler with HIV." In *Travel Medicine,* edited by J. S. Keystone, P. E. Kozarsky, D. O. Freedman, H. D. Nothdurft, and B. A. Connor. Edinburgh: Mosby, 2004: 241–47.

Castelli, I., and G. Carosi. "Epidemiology of Traveler's Diarrhea." *Chemotherapy* 41, suppl. 1 (1995): 20–32.

CDC web site on SARS: *http://www.cdc.gov/NCIDOD/SARS/*.

Chen, L., M. Wilson, and P. Schlagenhauf. "Prevention of Malaria in Long-Term Travelers." *Journal of the American Medical Association* 296, no. 18 (November 8, 2006): 2234–44.

Collins, K. J. "Heat Stress and Associated Disorders." In *Manson's Tropical Diseases*, edited by G. C. Cook and A. I. Zumla, 21st ed. London: W. B. Saunders, 2003: 545.

Cook, G. C., and A. I. Zumla, eds. *Manson's Tropical Diseases*, 21st ed. London: W. B. Saunders, 2003.

Cornall, P., S. Howie, A. Mughal, V. Sumner, F. Dunstan, A. Kemp, and J. Sibert. "Drowning of British Children Abroad." *Child Care and Health Development* 5 (September 31, 2005): 611–13.

Cortés, L. M., S. W. Hargarten, and H. M. Hennes. "Recommendations for Water Safety and Drowning Prevention for Travelers." *Journal of Travel Medicine* 13, no. 1 (January–February 2006): 21–34.

De Schryver, A., and A. Meheus. "International Travel and Sexually Transmitted Diseases." *World Health Statistics Quarterly* 42, no. 2 (1989): 90–99.

Delfino, R. J., R. S. Zeiger, J. M. Seltzer, et al. "Associations of Asthma Symptoms with Peak Particulate Air Pollution and Effect Modification by Anti-Inflammatory Medication Use." *Environmental Health Perspectives* 110, no. 10 (2002): A607–17.

Dematte, J. E., K. O'Mara, J. Bueschler, et al. "Near-Fatal Heat Stroke during the 1995 Heat Wave in Chicago." *Annals of Internal Medicine* 129 (1998): 173–81.

Dickey, J. H. "No Room to Breathe: Air Pollution and Primary Care Medicine. A Project of Greater Boston PSR (Physicians for Social Responsibility)." *http://www.psr.org/ breathe.htm*.

Dockery, D. W., C. A. Pope, X. Xu, et al. "An Association between

Air Pollution and Mortality in Six US Cities." *New England Journal of Medicine* 329, no. 24 (1993): 1807–8.

DuPont, H. L., and C. D. Ericsson. "Prevention and Treatment of Traveler's Diarrhea." *New England Journal of Medicine* 328 (1993): 1821–27.

DuPont, H. L., C. D. Ericsson, P. C. Johnson, J. A. Bitsura, M. W. DuPont, and F. J. de la Cabada. "Prevention of Traveler's Diarrhea by the Tablet Formulation of Bismuth Subsalicylate." *Journal of the American Medical Association* 257 (1987): 1347–50.

DuPont, H. L., and R. Steffen, eds. *Textbook of Travel Medicine and Health*, 2nd ed. Hamilton, ON: B. C. Decker Inc., 2001.

Durrheim, D. N., and J. M. Govere. "Malaria Outbreak Control in an African Village by Community Application of 'Deet' Mosquito Repellent to Ankles and Feet." *Medical and Veterinary Entomology* 16 (2002): 112–15.

Durrheim, D. N., and P. A. Leggat. "Risk to Tourists Posed by Wild Mammals in South Africa." *Journal of Travel Medicine* 6, no. 3 (September 1999): 172–79.

Eichmann, A. "Sexually Transmissible Diseases Following Travel in Tropical Countries." (In German.) *Schweiz Med Wochenschr* 123, no. 24 (1993): 1250–55.

Ericsson, C. D. "Travelers' Diarrhea. Epidemiology, Prevention, and Self-Treatment." *Infectious Disease Clinics of North America* 12 (1998): 285–303.

Ericsson, C. D., H. L. DuPont, and R. Steffen, eds. *Travelers' Diarrhea*. Hamilton, ON: B. C. Decker Inc., 2003.

Faucher, J. F., R. Binder, M. A. Missinou, P. B. Matsiegui, H. Gruss, R. Neubauer, B. Lell, J. U. Que, G. B. Miller, and P. G. Kremsner. "Efficacy of Atovaquone/Proguanil for Malaria Prophylaxis in Children and Its Effect on the Immunogenicity of Live Oral Typhoid and Cholera Vaccines." *Clinical Infectious Diseases* 35 (2002): 1147–54.

Forjuoh, S. N., C. N. Mock, D. I. Freidman, and R. Quansah. "Transport of the Injured to Hospitals in Ghana: The Need to Strengthen the Practice of Trauma Care." *Pre-hosp Immediate Care* 3 (1999): 66–70.

Fradin, M. S. "Mosquitoes and Mosquito Repellents: A Clinician's Guide." *Annals of Internal Medicine* 128, 11 (June 1, 1998): 931–40.

Franz, C., L. Havens, and S. Rogers, eds. *The People's Guide to Mexico: Wherever You Go . . . There You Are!!* Santa Fe, NM: John Muir Publications, 1998.

Freese, B. *Coal: A Human History.* Cambridge, MA: Perseus Publishing, 2003: 1.

Giovanetti, F. "Travel Medicine Interventions and Neurological Disease." *Travel Medicine and Infectious Disease* 5, no. 1 (January 2007): 7–17.

Goldsmid, J. M., S. S. Bettiol, and N. Sharples. "A Preliminary Study on Health Issues of Medical Students Undertaking Electives." *Journal of Travel Medicine* 10 (2003): 160–63.

Govere, J., L. E. Braack, D. N. Durrheim, R. H. Hunt, and M. Coetzee. "Repellent Effects on *Anopheles arabiensis* Biting Humans in Kruger Park, South Africa." *Medical and Veterinary Entomology* 15 (2001): 287–92.

Guerrant, R. L., D. H. Walker, and P. F. Weller, eds. *Tropical Infectious Diseases: Principles, Pathogens, and Practice.* Philadelphia: Churchill Livingston, 1999.

Guptill, K. S., S. W. Hargarten, and T. D. Baker. "American Travel Deaths in Mexico: Causes and Prevention Strategies." *Western Journal of Medicine* 154, no. 2 (1991): 169–71.

Guse, C. E., L. M. Cortes, S. W. Hargarten, and H. M. Hennes. "Injury Deaths to US Citizens Abroad." Injury and Violence in America Conference, Denver, May 10, 2005.

Halioua, B., T. Prazuck, and J. E. Malkin. "Sexually Transmitted

Diseases and Travel." (In French.) *Médecine tropicale* 57, no. 4 (March 1997): 501–4.

Hargarten, S. W., T. D. Baker, and K. Guptill. "Overseas Fatalities of United States Citizen Travelers: An Analysis of Deaths Related to International Travel." *Annals of Emergency Medicine* 20, no. 6 (1991): 622–26.

Hargarten, S. W., and G. T. Bouc. "Emergency Air Medical Transport of US Citizen Tourists: 1988–90." *Air Medical Journal* 12 (1993): 398–402.

Hargarten, S. W., and L. Mass. "Injury Fatalities to International Travelers: An Endemic Problem." Fifth World Conference in Injury Prevention, New Delhi, March 5–8, 2000.

Harris, A. F., A. Matias-Arnez, and N. Hill. "Biting Time of *Anopheles darlingi* in the Bolivian Amazon and Implications for Control of Malaria." *Transactions of the Royal Society of Tropical Medicine and Hygiene* 100 (2006): 45–47.

"Heat-Related Deaths—Chicago, Illinois, 1996–2001, and United States, 1979–1999." *Morbidity and Mortality Weekly Report* 51, no. 26: 567–70.

Hedley, A. J., C. M. Wong, T. Q. Thach, et al. "Cardiorespiratory and All-Cause Mortality after Restrictions on Sulphur Content of Fuel in Hong Kong: An Intervention Study." *Lancet* 360 (2002): 1646–52.

Herold, E. S., and C. Van Kerkwijk. "AIDS and Sex Tourism." *AIDS and Society* 4, no. 1 (1992): 1–8.

Hill, D. R., and R. H. Behrens. "A Survey of Travel Clinics throughout the World." *Journal of Travel Medicine* 3 (1996): 46–51.

Hill, D. R., C. D. Ericsson, R. D. Pearson, J. S. Keystone, D. O. Freedman, P. E. Kozarsky, H. L. DuPont, F. J. Bia, P. R. Fischer, and E. T. Ryan. "The Practice of Travel Medicine: Guidelines by the Infectious Diseases Society of America." *Clinical Infectious Diseases* 43, no. 12 (December 15, 2006): 1499–539. Epub. November 8, 2006.

Hombach, J., A. D. Barrett, M. J. Cardose, et al. "Review on Flavivirus Vaccine Development: Proceedings of a Meeting Jointly Organized by the World Health Organization and the Thai Ministry of Public Health, 26–27 April 2004, Bangkok, Thailand." *Vaccine* 23 (2005): 2689–95.

Hughes, C., R. Tucker, B. Bannister, and D. J. Bradley. "Malaria Prophylaxis for Long-Term Travelers." *Communicable Disease and Public Health.* Health Protection Agency Advisory Committee on Malaria Prevention for UK Travelers (ACMP) 6 (2003): 200–208.

"Insect Repellents: Which Keep Bugs at Bay?" *Consumer Reports* (June 2006): 6.

"Islands in the (Air) Stream." *Science@NASA. http://science.msfc.nasa.gov/newhome/headlines/essd01may98_1.htm.*

Jelinek, T., G. Dobler, M. Holscher, et al. "Prevalence of Infection with Dengue Virus among International Travelers." *Archives of Internal Medicine* 157, no. 20 (1997): 2367–70.

Jong, E. C., and C. Sanford, eds. *The Travel and Tropical Medicine Manual,* 4th ed. Philadelphia: Saunders/Elsevier, 2008.

Jong, E. C., and J. N. Zuckerman, eds. *Travelers' Vaccines.* Hamilton, ON: B. C. Decker Inc., 2004.

Just, J., C. Segala, F. Sahraoui, et al. "Short-Term Health Effects of Particulate and Photochemical Air Pollution in Asthmatic Children." *European Respiratory Journal* 20, no. 4 (2002): 899–906.

Kaiser, R., C. H. Rubin, A. K. Henderson, et al. "Heat-Related Death and Mental Illness during the 1999 Cincinnati Heat Wave." *American Journal of Forensic Medicine and Pathology* 22, no. 3 (2001): 303–7.

Keystone, J. S., P. E. Kozarsky, D. O. Freedman, H. D. Nothdurft, and B. A. Connor, eds. *Travel Medicine.* Edinburgh: Mosby, 2004.

Kolb, C., S. Schmieder, G. Lehmann, B. Zrenner, M. R. Karch, A. Plewan, and C. Schmitt. "Do Airport Metal Detectors Interfere with Implantable Pacemakers or Cardioverter-Defibrillators?"

Journal of American College of Cardiology 41, no. 11 (June 4, 2003): 2054–59.

Koutsky, L. A., K. A. Ault, C. M. Wheeler, D. R. Brown, E. Barr, F. B. Alvarez, L. M. Chiacchierini, and K. U. Jansen. "A Controlled Trial of a Human Papillomavirus Type 16 Vaccine." Proof of Principle Study Investigators. *New England Journal of Medicine* 347, no. 21 (November 21, 2002): 1645–51.

Krakauer, Jon. *Into Thin Air: A Personal Account of the Mt. Everest Disaster.* New York: Villard, 1977.

Krug, E., ed. "Injury: A Leading Cause of the Global Burden of Disease." Geneva: WHO, 1999. *http://www.who.int/violence_injury _prevention/index.html.*

Kunii, O., S. Kanagawa, I. Yajima, et al. "The 1997 Haze Disaster in Indonesia: Its Air Quality and Health Effects." *Archives of Environmental Health* 57, no. 1 (2002): 16–22.

Kuschner, R. A., A. F. Trofa, R. J. Thomas, et al. "Use of Azithromycin for the Treatment of Campylobacter Enteritis in Travelers to Thailand, an Area Where Ciprofloxacin Resistance Is Prevalent." *Clinical Infectious Diseases* 21 (1995): 536–41.

Kusumi, R. D. "Medical Aspects of Air Travel." *American Family Physician* 23, no. 6 (1981): 125–29.

Kyriacou, D. N., E. L. Arcinue, C. Peek, and J. F. Kraus. "Effect of Immediate Resuscitation on Children with Submersion Injury." *Pediatrics* 94 (1994): 137–42.

Layton, M. L., and F. J. Bia. "Emerging Issues in Travel Medicine." *Current Opinion in Infectious Diseases* 5 (1992): 338–44.

Leggat, P. A., J. L. Heydon, and A. Menon. "Health Advice Given by General Practitioners for Travelers from New Zealand." *New Zealand Medical Journal* 112, no. 1087 (1999): 158–61.

Leggat, P. A., and M. Klein. "Personal Safety Advice for Travelers Abroad." *Journal of Travel Medicine* 8 (2001): 46–51.

Leithead, C. S., and A. R. Lind. *Heat Stress and Heat Disorders*. London: Cassell, 1964.

Lillie, T. H., C. E. Schreck, and A. J. Rahe. "Effectiveness of Personal Protection against Mosquitoes in Alaska." *Journal of Medical Entomology* 25 (1988): 475–78.

Lind, J. *An Essay on Diseases Incidental to Europeans in Hot Climates*. London: T. Becket, 1768.

Luxemburger, C., R. N. Price, and F. Nosten. "Mefloquine in Infants and Young Children." *Annals of Tropical Paediatrics* 16 (1996): 281.

MacCannell, D. *The Tourist: A New Theory of the Leisure Class*. Berkeley: University of California Press, 1999.

Mackell, S. M. "Vaccinations for the Pediatric Traveler." *Clinical Infectious Diseases* 37 (2003): 1508.

MacPherson, D. W., D. L. Guerillot, K. Streinter, et al. "Death and Dying Abroad: The Canadian Experience." *Journal of Travel Medicine* 7 (2000): 227–33.

Maire, N., J. J. Aponte, A. Ross, R. Thompson, P. Alonso, J. Utzinger, M. Tanner, and T. Smith. "Modeling a Field Trial of the RTS,S/AS02A Malaria Vaccine." *American Journal of Tropical Medicine and Hygiene* 75, suppl. 2 (August 2006): 104–10.

Manchester, W. *Last Lion: Winston Spencer Churchill: Alone, 1932–40*. Boston: Little, Brown & Co., 1978: 878.

Martin, M., L. H. Weld, and T. F. Tsai. "Advanced Age as a Risk Factor for Illness Temporally Associated with Yellow Fever Vaccination." *Emerging Infectious Disease* 7 (2001): 945–51.

McCarthy, A. E. "Travelers with Pre-existing Disease." In *Travel Medicine*, edited by J. S. Keystone, P. E. Kozarsky, D. O. Freedman, H. D. Nothdurft, and B. A. Connor. Edinburgh: Mosby, 2004:

McLellan, Susan. "Travel and HIV Infection." In Jong and Sanford, eds., *The Travel and Tropical Medicine Manual*, 4th ed. Philadelphia: Saunders/Elsevier, 2008.

McConnell, R., K. Berhane, F. Gilliland, et al. "Asthma in Exercising Children Exposed to Ozone: A Cohort Study." *Lancet* 359 (2002): 386–91.

The Medical Letter on Drugs and Therapeutics 45 (July 21, 2003): 58–60.

The Medical Letter on Drugs and Therapeutics 46, no. 1191 (September 13, 2004) http://www.medicalletter.org, on Rifaximine.

Memish, Z. A. "Meningococcal Disease and Travel." *Clinical Infectious Diseases* 34 (2002): 84–90.

Mock, C. N., K. E. S. Adzotor, L. Conklin, D. M. Denno, and G.-Jurkovich. "Trauma Outcomes in the Rural Developing World: Comparison with an Urban Level I Trauma Center." *Journal of Trauma* 35 (1993): 518–23.

Mock, C. N., G. Asiamah, and J. Amegashie. "A Random, Roadside Breathalyzer Survey of Alcohol Impaired Driving in Ghana." *Journal of Crash Prevention & Injury Control* 2, no. 3 (2001): 193–202.

Mock, C. N., G. J. Jurkovich, and D. nii-Amon-Kotei. "Trauma Mortality Patterns in Three Nations at Different Economic Levels: Implications for Global Trauma System Development." *Journal of Trauma* 44 (1998): 804–14.

Monath, T. P. "Yellow Fever." In *Vaccines*, 3rd ed., edited by S. A. Plotkin and W. Orenstein. Philadelphia: W. B. Saunders, 1999: 858–63.

Monath, T. P., F. Guirakhoo, R. Nichols, et al. "Chimeric Live, Attenuated Vaccine against Japanese Encephalitis (ChimeriVax-JE): Phase 2 Clinical Trials for Safety and Immunogenicity, Effect of Vaccine Dose and Schedule, and Memory Response to Challenge with Inactivated Japanese Encephalitis Antigen." *Journal of Infectious Diseases* 188, no.8 (2003): 1213–30.

Moore, J., C. Beeker, J. S. Harrison, et al. "Risk Behavior among Peace Corps Volunteers." *AIDS* 9 (1995): 795–99.

Moore, S. J., A. Lenglet, and N. Hill. "Field Evaluation of Three

Plant-Based Insect Repellents against Malaria Vectors in Vaca Diez Province, the Bolivian Andes." *Journal of the American Mosquito Control Association* 18 (2002): 107–10.

Muentener, P., P. Schlagenhauf, and R. Steffen. "Imported Malaria (1985–95): Trends and Perspectives." *Bulletin of the World Health Organization* 77 (1999): 560–66.

Muhm, J. M., P. B. Rock, D. L. McMullin, et al. "Effect of Aircraft-Cabin Altitude on Passenger Discomfort." *New England Journal of Medicine* 357, no. 1 (2007): 18–27.

Mulhall, B. P., M. Hu, M. Thompson, et al. "Planned Sexual Behavior of Young Australian Visitors to Thailand." *Medical Journal of Australia* 158, no. 8 (1993): 530–35.

Murray, C., and A. Lopez. *The Global Burden of Disease.* Cambridge: Harvard University Press, 1996.

Murray, J. "Infection as a Cause of Multiple Sclerosis." *British Medical Journal* 325 (2002): 1128.

Mutsch, M., M. Tavernini, A. Marx, V. Gregory, Y. P. Lin, A. J. Hay, A. Tschopp, and R. Steffen. "Influenza Virus Infection in Travelers to Tropical and Subtropical Countries." *Clinical Infectious Diseases* 40, no. 9 (May 1, 2005): 1282–87. Epub. March 28, 2005.

Nantulya, V. M., and F. K. Muli-Musiime. "Uncovering the Social Determinants of Road Traffic Accidents." In *Challenging Inequities: From Ethics to Action,* edited by T. Evans, M. Whitehead, F. Diderichsen, et al. Oxford: Oxford University Press, 2001: 211–25.

Nasci, R. "Pre- and Post-Travel General Health Recommendations: Protection against Mosquitoes and Other Arthropods." In *Health Information for International Travelers, 2005–6,* edited by P. M. Arguin, P. E. Kozarsky, and A. W. Navin. Atlanta: US Dept. of Health and Human Services, Public Health Service, 2005:24–28.

National Highway Traffic Safety Administration (NHTSA). *Traffic*

Safety Facts, 1999. http://www.nhtsa.dot.gov/people/ncsa/pdf/TSF0
vr99.R.pdf.

Newton, P. N., R. McGready, F. Fernandez, et al. "Manslaughter
by Fake Artesunate in Asia—Will Africa Be Next?" *PLoS Medicine* 2006: 197.

Ng'walali, P. M., A. Koreeda, K. Kibayashi, and S. Tsunenari.
"Fatalities by Inhalation of Volcanic Gas at Mt. Aso Crater in
Kumamoto, Japan." *Journal of Legal Medicine* (Tokyo) 1, no. 3
(September 1999): 180–84.

Noble, S. L., E. Johnston, and B. Walton. "Insulin Lispro: A Fast-
Acting Insulin Analog." *American Family Physician* 57, no. 2 (January 15, 1998): 279–86, 289–92.

Nothdurft, H. D., T. Jelinek, S. M. Pechel, et al. "Stand-By Treatment
of Suspected Malaria in Travelers." *Tropical Medicine and Parasi-
tology* 46 (1995): 161–63.

Ostro, B. D., G. S. Eskeland, J. M. Sanchez, and T. Feyzioglu. "Air
Pollution and Health Effects: A Study of Medical Visits among
Children in Santiago, Chile." *Environmental Health Perspectives*
107, no. 1 (1999): 69–73.

Page, S. J., and D. Meyer. "Tourist Accidents." *Annals of Tourism
Research* 23 (1996): 666–90.

Paixao, M. L. T., R. D. Dewar, J. H. Cossar, et al. "What Do Scots
Die of When Abroad?" *Scottish Medical Journal* 36 (1991): 114–16.

Petridou, E., H. Askitopoulou, D. Vourvahakis, et al. "Epidemiology of Road Traffic Accidents during Pleasure Traveling: The
Evidence from the Island of Crete." *Accident; Analysis and Prevention* 29 (1997): 687–93.

Petridou, E., N. Dessypris, A. Skalkidou, et al. "Are Traffic Injuries Disproportionally More Common among Tourists in
Greece? Struggling with Incomplete Data." *Accident; Analysis
and Prevention* 31, no. 6 (1999): 611–15.

"Please Slow Down." *The Economist* (February 7, 2002): 46.

Plotkin, S. A., W. A. Orenstein, and P. A. Offit. *Vaccines*, 4th ed. Philadelphia: W. B. Saunders, 2003.

Pollard, A. J., S. Niermeyer, P. Barry, et al. "Children at High Altitude: An International Consensus Statement by an Ad Hoc Committee of the International Society for Mountain Medicine, March 12, 2001." *High Altitude Medicine & Biology* 2, no. 3 (Fall 2001): 389–403.

Pope, C. A., R. T. Burnett, M. J. Thun, et al. "Lung Cancer, Cardiopulmonary Mortality, and Long-Term Exposure to Fine Particulate Air Pollution." *Journal of the American Medical Association* 287, no. 9 (2002): 1132–41.

Potasman, I., A. Beny, and H. Seligmann. "Neuropsychiatric Problems in 2,500 Long-Term Young Travelers to the Tropics." *Journal of Travel Medicine* 7, no. 5 (2000): 225–26.

Prociv, P. "Deaths of Australian Travelers Overseas." *Medical Journal of Australia* 163 (1995): 27–30.

Pro-MED. "Measles Eradication—Worldwide: New Targets." January 25, 2007. http://www.promedmail.org.

Rajpal, R. C., M. G. Weisskopf, P. D. Rumm, et al. "Wisconsin, July 1999 Heat Wave: An Epidemiologic Assessment." *Journal of Wilderness Medicine* 99, no. 5 (2000): 41–44.

Salifu, M., and C. N. Mock. "Pedestrian Injuries in Kumasi: Results of an Epidemiological Survey." *Ghana Engineer* 18 (1998): 23–27.

Sanford, C. "Urban Medicine: Threats to Health of Travelers to Developing World Cities." *Journal of Travel Medicine* 11 (September–October 2004): 313–27.

Sanford, C., ed. *Primary Care Clinics: Travel Medicine.* Philadelphia: Saunders/Elsevier, 2002.

Schlagenhauf, P., ed. *Travelers' Malaria.* Hamilton, ON: B. C. Decker Inc., 2001.

Schlagenhauf, P., R. Steffen, A. Tschopp, et al. "Behavioural Aspects of Travelers in Their Use of Malaria Presumptive

Treatment." *Bulletin of the World Health Organization* 73 (1995): 215–21.

Schwartz, E., E. Mendelson, and Y. Sidi. "Dengue Fever among Travelers." *American Journal of Medicine* 101, no. 5 (1996): 516–20.

Sejvar, J., E. Bancroft, K. Winthrop, J. Bettinger, M. Bajani, S. Bragg, K. Shutt, R. Kaiser, N. Marano, T. Popovic, J. Tappero, D. Ashford, L. Mascola, D. Vugia, B. Perkins, and N. Rosenstein. "Eco-Challenge Investigation Team. Leptospirosis in 'Eco-Challenge' Athletes, Malaysian Borneo, 2000." *Emerging Infectious Diseases* 9, no. 6 (June 2003): 702–7.

Stauffer, W. M., and D. Kamat. "Traveling with Infants and Young Children. Part III: Travelers' Diarrhea." *Journal of Travel Medicine* 9 (2002): 141.

Stauffer, W. M., D. Kamat, and A. J. Magill. "Traveling with Infants and Children. Part IV: Insect Avoidance and Malaria Prevention." *Journal of Travel Medicine* 10 (2003): 225.

Steffen, R. "Epidemiologic Studies of Traveler's Diarrhea, Severe Gastrointestinal Infections, and Cholera." *Reviews of Infectious Diseases* 8, suppl. 2 (1986): S122–30.

Steffen, R. "Travel Medicine—Prevention Based on Epidemiological Data." *Transactions of the Royal Society of Tropical Medicine and Hygiene* 85, no. 2 (1991): 156–62.

Steffen, R., N. Tornieporth, S. A. Clemens, S. Chatterjee, A. M. Cavalcanti, F. Collard, N. De Clercq, H. L. DuPont, and F. von Sonnenburg. "Epidemiology of Travelers' Diarrhea: Details of a Global Survey." *Journal of Travel Medicine* 11, no. 4 (July–August 2004): 231–37.

Steinberg, E. B., R. Bishop, P. Haber, A. F. Dempsey, R. M. Hoekstra, J. M. Nelson, M. Ackers, A. Calugar, and E. D. Mintz. "Typhoid Fever in Travelers: Who Should Be Targeted for Prevention?" *Clinical Infectious Diseases* 39, no. 2 (July 15, 2004): 186–91.

Strickland, G. T., ed. *Hunter's Tropical Medicine and Emerging Infectious Diseases*, 8th ed. Philadelphia: W. B. Saunders, 2000.

Strum, W. B. "Update on Traveler's Diarrhea." *Journal of Postgraduate Medicine* 84, no. 1 (1988): 163–66, 169–70.

Sudhir, P., and C. E. Prasad. "Prevalence of Exercise-Induced Bronchospasm in Schoolchildren: An Urban-Rural Comparison." *Journal of Tropical Pediatrics* 49, no. 2 (2003): 104–8.

Suh, K. N., and M. D. Meleno. "Challenging Scenarios in a Travel Clinic: Advising the Complex Traveler." *Infectious Disease Clinics of North America* 18, no. 1 (March 2005).

Tattevin, P., A. G. Depatureaux, and J. M. Chapplain. "Yellow Fever Vaccine is Safe and Effective in HIV-Infected Patients." *AIDS* 18 (2004): 835–37.

Tauber, E., H. Kollartisch, M. Korinek, et al. "Safety and Immunogenicity of a Vero-cell Derived, Inactivated Japanese Encephalitis Vaccine: A Non-inferiority, Phase III, Randomized Controlled Trial." *Lancet* 370 (2007): 1847–53.

Tauxe, R. V., and J. M. Hughes. "Food-Borne Disease." In *Douglas and Bennett's Principles and Practice of Infectious Diseases*, edited by G. L. Mandell, J. E. Bennett, and R. Dolin, 4th ed. New York: Churchill Livingstone, 1995: 1012–24.

Taylor, L. H., S. M. Latham, and M. E. Woolhouse. "Risk Factors for Human Disease Emergence." *Philosophical Transactions: Biological Sciences* 356, no. 1411 (2001): 983–89.

Theis, M. K., B. Honigman, R. Yip, D. McBride, C. S. Houston, and L. G. Moore. "Acute Mountain Sickness in Children at 2835 Meters." *Archives of Pediatrics & Adolescent Medicine* 147, no. 2 (February 1993).

Thompson, D. T., D. V. Ashley, C. A. Dockery-Brown, et al. "Incidence of Health Crises in Tourists Visiting Jamaica, West Indies, 1998–2000." *Journal of Travel Medicine* 10, no. 2 (2003): 79–86.

United Nations Economic and Social Commission for Asia and the Pacific. http://www.unescap.org/enrd/ environment/activities/ES/ SOE/CH06.PDF.

United States Department of Health and Human Services. The National Women's Health Information Center. "Pregnancy and Medicine." http://www.womenshealth.gov/faq/pregmed.htm.

United States Department of State, Bureau of Consular Affairs. February 2000. http://www.state.gov.

United States Drug Enforcement Agency. "The Changing Face of European Drug Policy." Drug Intelligence Brief (April 2002). http:// www.dea.gov.

United States Food and Drug Administration (FDA). "FDA Licenses New Vaccine for Prevention of Cervical Cancer and Other Diseases in Females Caused by Human Papillomavirus." News release. http://www.fda.gov/bbs/topics/NEWS/2006/NEW01385.html.

"Update: Leptospirosis and Unexplained Acute Febrile Illness among Athletes Participating in Triathlons—Illinois and Wisconsin, 1998." Morbidity and Mortality Weekly Report 47, no. 32 (August 21, 1998): 673–76.

Van Herck, K., J. Zuckerman, F. Castelli, et al. "Travelers' Knowledge, Attitudes, and Practices on Prevention of Infectious Diseases: Results from a Pilot Study." Journal of Travel Medicine 10 (2003): 75–78.

Velasco, M., S. Morote, C. Aramburu, et al. "Sexual Behavior Risk in Spanish International Travelers." Medicina clínica 116, no. 16 (2001): 612–13.

Warrell, D. A., and H. M. Gilles, eds. Essential Malariology, 4th ed. London: Arnold, 2002.

Waterhouse, J., T. Reilly, G. Atkinson, and B. Edwards. "Jet Lag: Trends and Coping Strategies." Lancet 369, no. 9567 (March 31, 2007): 1117–29.

Wolfson, L. J., P. M. Strebel, M. Gacic-Dobo, E. J. Hoekstra, J. W.

McFarland, and B. S. Hersh. "Measles Initiative: Has the 2005 Measles Mortality Reduction Goal Been Achieved? A Natural History Modelling Study." *Lancet* 369, no. 9557 (January 20, 2007): 191–200.

World Bank Group. "World Development Indicators 2007." http://www.worldbank.org/data/wdi2002/pdfs/table%203–13.pdf.

World Health Organization (WHO). "Cumulative Number of Confirmed Human Cases of Avian Influenza A/(H5N1) Reported to WHO." February 3, 2007. http://www.who.int/csr/disease/avian_influenza/country/cases_table_2007_02_03/en/index.html.

World Health Organization (WHO). "Disease Outbreaks Reported, May 8, 2002. Dengue/Dengue Haemorrhagic Fever in Brazil—Update 2." WHO: Communicable Disease Surveillance and Response. http://www.who.int/ disease-outbreak-news/n2002/may/8may2002.html (accessed August 2, 2003).

World Health Organization (WHO). "Malaria." In *International Travel and Health*. Geneva: WHO, 2005: 132–51. http://whqlibdoc.who.int/publications/2005/9241580364_chap7.pdf.

Yaron, M., S. Niermeyer, K. N. Lindgren, and B. Honigman. "Evaluation of Diagnostic Criteria and Incidence of Acute Mountain Sickness in Preverbal Children." *Wilderness & Environmental Medicine* 13, no. 1 (Spring 2002): 21–26.

Yozwiak, S. "Island Sizzle: Growth May Make Valley an Increasingly Hot Spot." *Arizona Republic* (September 25, 1998).

About the Author

Christopher Sanford is a family practice physician who specializes in travel and tropical medicine. He earned a master of public health degree at the Harvard School of Public Health; a Diploma in Tropical Medicine & Hygiene from Universidad Peruana Cayetano Heredia in Lima, Peru; an MD from the University of California, San Diego; a BA in psychology from the University of California, Santa Barbara; and no degree from El Camino College in Torrance, California, despite two and a half years of sincere socializing. He completed a residency in family practice at San Jose Medical Center/ Stanford University (now San Jose-O'Connor Hospital Family Medicine Residency Program), and has been awarded a Certificate of Knowledge in Clinical Tropical Medicine & Travelers' Health from the American Society of Tropical Medicine & Hygiene. He is board certified in family practice. Currently Dr. Sanford serves as co-director of the University of Washington Travel Clinic at Hall Health Center. He also practices travel medicine at Boeing's International Health Services. He lives in Seattle with his wife and two sons.

The field of travel medicine, encompassing as it does all illnesses and manner of injury in all nations, is too vast for any one person to master. If you have suggestions, additions, or corrections, please drop me a line at:

Christopher Sanford
c/o University of Washington Press
P.O. Box 50096
Seattle, WA 98145–5096
USA

or

sanford99@gmail.com

Index

lack of knowledge in, 9; time frame for visits to, 6; topics discussed during appointments with, 7–9

prednisone, 73, 134

pregnancy and anti-malarials, 54–55

prescriptions, 155

pressure stockings, 163

prevention: of altitude illnesses, 142; of drowning, 70; insect avoidance, 42–47, 135; of road traffic accidents, 67–69

primaquine, 57–58

prions, 150

prochlorperazine (Compazine), 141

promethazine (Phenergan), 112–113

psychosis, 60

pulmonary disease, 72–73

pulmonary edema, 123

pyelonephritis, 105

Qinghaosu, 61–62

rabies, 32–34, 117–118

reduviid bugs, 150

renal failure, 133

Repel oil of lemon eucalyptus, 46

resources for travelers: associa-

tions, 180; conferences, 180–181; guides, 178; medical-related books, 177–178; online, 178–179

responsible traveling, 176

retinal damage, 53

rifaximin (Xifaxan), 101, 132

robbery, 77

RotaTeq (rotavirus vaccine), 115

rotavirus, 115

Royal Society of Tropical Medicine and Hygiene (RSTMH), 180

rubella, 12–13, 114, 131

Sabah, 88

safety: for children, 111, 119; in game parks, 152; at high elevations, 142–143; in traffic, 67–69; around volcanoes, 151

salicylates, 118

Salmonella, 94, 104

SARS, 91

Saudi Arabia, 27

schistosomiasis (bilharzia), 122, 167–168

scopolamine, 113

scuba diving, 9

seat belts, 8, 67, 69

security, 8

sedatives, 142

seizures, 52